# MUSCULOSKELETAL DISORDERS
## COMMON PROBLEMS

*To Chris*

*Congratulations and best wishes always,*

*Barbara M. Edwardson*

## Barbara M. Edwardson, M.Ed.
Professor Emerita
Department of Physical Therapy
Faculty of Applied Health Sciences
The University of Western Ontario
London, Ontario
Canada

## SINGULAR PUBLISHING GROUP, INC.
San Diego, California

Singular Publishing Group, Inc.
4284 41st Street
San Diego, California 92105-1197

©1995 by Singular Publishing Group, Inc.

Typeset in 10/12 New Century Schoolbook by SoCal Graphics
Printed in the Untied States of America by McNaughton & Gunn

**Library of Congress Cataloging-in-Publication data**
Edwardson, Barbara M., 1929–
   Musculoskeletal disorders : common problems / Barbara M.
Edwardson.
     p.    cm.
   Includes bibliographical references and index.
   ISBN 1-56593-170-X
   1. Musculoskeletal system—Diseases—Physical therapy.    I. Title.
   [DNLM: 1. Musculoskeletal Diseases—therapy. 2. Musculoskeletal
Diseases—diagnosis. 3. Physical Therapy.  WE  140 E26m  1994]
   RC925.5.E39  1994
   616.7—dc20
   DNLM/DLC
   for Library of Congress               94-31570
                                      CIP

# CONTENTS

# FOREWORD

Musculoskeletal disease in its almost countless forms has been slowly defined in the last 50 years. Precise disease classification criteria have become more relevant as physical therapy has become less empirical. This knowledge has led to the application of specific treatment strategies designed to influence, not just impairments, but also levels of disability. We are informed that physical therapy is on the threshold of an excitingly different era. The knowledge is there, and the physical therapies are now being tested.

This unique book, by a well-known academic physical therapist, recognizes the crucial importance of being able accurately to assess musculoskeletal conditions, develop treatment plans, and judge the outcomes of physical therapy. A previous book by Professor Edwardson, *Musculoskeletal Assessment: An Integrated Approach*, has covered the basics of musculoskeletal assessments.

Professor Edwardson has carefully mapped out the subject of this book so that readers, students, and physical therapists alike can progress logically and on a regional basis from the underlying structure and function of each segment to its pathophysiology, symptomatology, and treatment. This book will also provide indispensable resource material for educators of the musculoskeletal diseases and others with an interest in this subject.

To be asked by Professor Edwardson to write a foreword for *Musculoskeletal Disorders: Common Problems* has been a distinct honor.

Antoine Helewa
Professor and Chair
Department of Physical Therapy
University of Western Ontario
London, Ontario, Canada

# PREFACE

This book has evolved over many years of teaching courses on musculoskeletal assessment and musculoskeletal disorders to second and third year students of physical therapy at the University of Western Ontario, Canada. Much of what is contained here is a response to their questions and suggestions; it is therefore a text primarily written for physical therapy students and new graduates, although other members of the health care professions will find it helpful.

The conditions and related aspects discussed represent **some** of those commonly encountered by physical therapists in their dealing with adult musculoskeletal disorders. Pediatric problems are not presented, nor are the arthritides, apart from degenerative processes of the spine and the hip joint.

The subject matter associated with musculoskeletal disorders is extensive and a knowledge of anatomy and biomechanical principles is fundamental to an understanding of these disorders. Consequently each chapter begins with a review of the pertinent anatomy, which will help the reader's orientation to the subject matter under discussion.

Because every patient is different and therapists' preferences for particular treatment approaches vary, I have, except in a few instances, avoided specific treatment programs, resorting instead to treatment guidelines. References are provided throughout so that the reader can pursue established treatment procedures and further detail regarding the subject matter.

The book is divided into 11 chapters. Chapter 1, the introductory chapter, introduces some of the common findings and basic principles relating to musculoskeletal disorders. Chapter 2 discusses common problems of the cervical spine and Chapter 3 focuses upon the shoulder girdle mechanism and associated problems. Chapter 4 involves conditions of the elbow, wrist, and hand, and Chapter 5 deals with conditions of the back region. Chapter 6 presents an introduction to the McKenzie approach to problems involving the low back region. Chapter 7 presents some insight into conditions in the region of the hip joint and Chapter 8 involves conditions related to the patellofemoral joint. Chapter 9 evolves around problems associated with the tibiofemoral joint and its passive structures. Chapter 10 contains information regarding foot and ankle problems. The final chapter, Chapter 11, introduces the reader to some basic facts relating to fractures.

The information contained in this book constitutes a beginning to what I hope will be an ongoing study on the part of the reader.

# ACKNOWLEDGMENTS

I am indebted to Sally Morgan for her painstaking editing of this manuscript and for her assistance and support in many other ways, and to Pat Darling for assuming the secretarial responsibilities with dedication and for keeping me calm at times of stress; without the contributions of these two members of the team this book may never have been completed. A special thanks to Janet Brown who undertook the task of illustrator at the eleventh hour and who did a magnificent job, to Tom Rush who volunteered his services as consultant for the computerized illustrations, and to Sue Morgan for her fine contribution to the illustrations. Finally, I am indebted to all my students over the years who have given this book its reason for being.

# CHAPTER 1

● ● ● ● ● ● ● ●

# Basic Principles

In this introductory chapter a number of aspects of musculoskeletal disorders will be discussed, beginning with a classification of the disorders.

## CLASSIFICATION OF MUSCULOSKELETAL DISORDERS

Musculoskeletal disorders consist of a number of conditions which may be grouped under different headings.

### Soft Tissue Injuries

Injuries to soft tissue implicate the tendons, muscles, ligaments, and related areas. The mechanism of injury can be traumatic, sustained during occupational or athletic activities, or it can be the result of a blow or fall. Overuse or repetitive stress are also mechanisms which commonly affect the soft tissues of the body. Prominent among the soft tissue injuries are those which result in inflammation of tendons (tendinitis), partial or complete rupture of a tendon, varying degrees of ligamentous sprain, strain or partial to complete rupture of muscle, and damage to blood vessels, nerve roots, and peripheral nerves.

## Degenerative Conditions

Degenerative conditions may involve soft tissue structures, but the term generally relates to joints of the spine and peripheral joints.

Degenerative conditions of the spine are fairly common and frequently commence with degenerative changes in the intervertebral disc. Cracks develop in the inner rings of the annulus fibrosus and the nuclear material leaks out through the cracks; this results in abnormal movement within the intervertebral joint and accompanying symptomatology. As the condition progresses the cracks extend to the outer rim of the annulus and bulging or protrusion of the disc occurs; the final stage is herniation when the nuclear material breaks through the outer rim of the annulus. With each progression of the degenerative condition of the disc there is an increase in symptomatology and involvement of the zygapophyseal joints which are intimately related to the intervertebral joint. Eventually not only will the intervertebral joint exhibit signs of degeneration, such as loss of joint space and osteophyte formation, but degenerative changes will also be evident in the zygapophyseal joints.

The peripheral joints affected by "wear and tear" degeneration are principally the weight bearing joints and in particular the hip and knee joints. Wear and tear develop as a result of excessive abnormal compression forces, usually on a vulnerable joint that has sustained a previous injury or is exhibiting abnormal mechanics. The articular cartilage is affected, resulting in degenerative changes that interfere with normal movement and give rise to pain as a result of stress on the sensitive soft tissue structures.

## Fractures and Dislocations

Fractures and dislocations are common injuries which usually develop as a result of direct or indirect violence sustained during an athletic activity or as a result of a fall. A fracture is a disruption in the normal contour of the cortical bone and a dislocation is a complete separation of the articular surfaces of a joint. In both types of injury the soft tissues are involved. Physical therapists, as a general rule, do not treat the fracture as such, but are very much involved in the treatment of the associated soft tissue damage and the resultant rehabilitation problems that are presented.

## Rheumatological Conditions

In addition to the conditions mentioned above there are a number of soft tissue and joint conditions that are grouped under the heading of rheumatology. These conditions commonly exhibit systemic symptoms and require specialized care from a medical specialist as well as from a physical therapist specializing in this area.

## Postural Problems and Asymmetries

Postural problems can develop in the spine or the peripheral joints and may be divided into those that are **non-structural** and those that are **structural**. The non-structural type of postural problem involves soft tissues and the condition is usually reversible by physical means; the structural type of postural problem involves soft tissue and bony structures and the changes are not reversible by physical means.

Asymmetries, some of which are present from birth, are a common finding in the musculoskeletal examination; for instance one bony point may be higher or lower than its partner on the opposite side or a muscle bulk may be larger on one side than the other. It is necessary for the physical therapist to note asymmetries; at the same time it is important to remember that from the time we become right- or left-sided dominant, asymmetries are going to develop naturally. They are only of significance if their presence is responsible for the patient's symptoms. This type of asymmetry can be detected from a thorough assessment of the patient.

## COMMON CLINICAL FINDINGS AND TREATMENT OBJECTIVES IN MUSCULOSKELETAL DISORDERS

In musculoskeletal disorders invariably one or more of the following clinical findings are treated, regardless of the condition. The most common finding is that of pain which is often the dominating symptom and the one which makes the patient seek help.

## Pain

Pain varies from an intermittent ache to a severe, unremitting, constant pain. It may be localized (found close to the site of injury) or referred (located some distance from the causative factor). The nature of the pain varies and may be described as stabbing, burning, throbbing and so on. The patient experiences pain as a result of stress, damage, deformation, or chemical irritation to structures containing nociceptor receptors. Pain is often associated with sensory disturbances such as numbness and paresthesia: for example a "pins and needles" sensation.

From the clinical viewpoint it is important for the therapist to determine: (a) whether the pain is constant or intermittent (severity), (b) the degree of irritability (how easily the pain increases in intensity and the length of time that increased intensity lasts), and (c) the nature of the pain described previously.

*Treatment Objective:* To locate the cause of the patient's pain and to reduce the activity of the nociceptor system by controlling the mechanism by which it is being enhanced.

## Muscle Weakness

In its simplest form weakness develops from lack of use—"what you don't use you lose." Clinically it can be caused by disuse resulting from a period of immobilization following a fracture or joint injury, or by pain as a result of trauma to a muscle component or involvement of nerve roots. Weakness can also be caused by damage to the peripheral nerves. In this case, as with damaged nerve roots, the weakness is usually more extensive and prolonged.

*Treatment Objective:* To restore normal extensibility, strength of contraction, and function to the muscle.

## Muscle Spasm

A painful stimulus can produce a prolonged, involuntary contraction of a muscle called muscle spasm. The spasm is protective in nature and serves to guard injured structures against adverse movement. However, although muscle spasm knows when to appear it does not always know when to disappear. Its presence is perpetuated by the obstruction of movement, causing muscle ischemia which causes pain resulting in further muscle spasm. When muscle spasm persists it can create other problems such as tightness of soft tissue structures, restriction of motion, and muscle weakness.

*Treatment Objectives:* To locate and treat the painful stimulus, induce relaxation of the muscles, and restore normal extensibility and function.

## Hypomobility

Essentially hypomobility is a loss of range of motion in a joint. It can result from a restriction of a **physiological** movement (the movement of the joint under the control of the patient): for example, restricted abduction of the glenohumeral joint. Restriction of a physiological movement will ultimately lead to restriction of motion of the accompanying **accessory** movement (the small articular movement over which the patient has no control): for instance, the inferior glide of the humeral head is the accompanying accessory motion to physiological abduction.

*Treatment Objective:* To identify the cause of the loss of movement and to restore normal range of motion and function.

## Instability

Excessive and uncontrolled movement develops as a result of damage to the stabilizing structures supporting the joint, for example, the ligaments. The medial aspect of the knee will demonstrate instability if the medial collateral ligament is completely torn; the excessive movement represents abduction of the tibia on the femur.

*Treatment Objectives:* To identify the damaged structure(s) and to utilize stabilizing treatment approaches (surgery is often necessary) to restore stability.

## Adaptive Shortening

Contractures develop in the soft tissues of the body, for instance, muscles, ligaments, and fascia. The tissues are habitually maintained in a shortened range; as a result the normal flexibility of the tissues is lost. Adaptive shortening can be a feature of the postural problems discussed previously.

*Treatment Objective:* To gently restore the normal flexibility of the tightened structures and to educate the patient so that recurrence of the problem will not take place.

## Compression Syndromes

Compression syndromes are not uncommon in the musculoskeletal system; they develop because one structure is compressing another, giving rise to an inflammatory response and pain. The compression can be intermittent, caused by a correctable biomechanical problem, or it can be sustained. Intermittent compression may arise from repetitive stress during which compression occurs repeatedly: for example, during the performance of certain activities, such as the "painful arc" in the performance of abduction of the glenohumeral joint. This is caused by compression of the coracoacromial arch on inflamed structures such as the supraspinatus. An example of sustained compression is a severe disc disorder in which nuclear material is compressing a nerve root(s). Under these circumstances surgical intervention may be warranted, particularly if there is no response to treatment by conservative means.

*Treatment Objectives:* To identify the cause of the compression and to employ a decompression treatment approach to the traumatized structure.

## Inflammatory Response

Inflammation represents the first stage in the process of healing (see later) and is a vascular response to injured tissue. The process is characterized by pain, heat, swelling, redness, and restriction of function.

*Treatment Objectives:* To control the inflammatory response to injury, and to prevent exacerbation and restore function.

## Swelling

Swelling is a characteristic of the inflammatory response described above. It can be exhibited by injured tendons (tendinitis), muscles (contusions), ligaments (sprains), and joints. There are two causes of swelling in a joint; one is synovitis involving the synovial membrane, with subsequent production of excess synovial fluid; the other is hemarthrosis (bleeding into the joint) which occurs in more severe joint injuries.

*Treatment Objectives:* To control the swelling as soon as possible before it becomes organized and causes interference with normal functioning of soft tissue structures.

The swelling in both synovitis and hemarthrosis stretches the joint capsule and compresses the capillaries contained within it. The consequent reduction of blood supply interferes with the normal exchange of substances between the joint capsule and the articular cartilage, predisposing the joint to degeneration. The enzymes in the blood serum and the leukocytes from the hemarthrosis cause destruction of the superficial layers of the cartilage (Cotta & Puhl, 1978).

## THE STAGES OF HEALING AND THEIR RELATIONSHIP TO TREATMENT APPROACHES

The first consideration in the treatment of an injured patient is the stage of healing presented. Each stage demands a different approach to treatment that must be respected if the normal functional level of the patient is to be restored as soon as possible. The three stages of healing of connective tissue are the same, regardless of the cause of the injury:

- inflammation—the acute stage;
- healing and repair—the subacute stage;
- remodelling—the chronic stage.

In the following description of the different stages each is assigned an **approximate** time period; it is important to remember that patients will respond differently because of their uniqueness, plus one stage overlaps to the next.

## The Stages of Healing

As indicated earlier there are three stages of healing.

### Inflammation

During the inflammation stage vascular changes are noted for the first 48 hours following tissue damage. Solutes and cells ooze out from the blood vessels, followed by clot formation. Early fibroblastic activity begins when neutralization of the chemical irritant has occurred and cellular debris has been removed by phagocytosis. This stage lasts 4–6 days. The signs of inflammation and the treatment objectives were noted previously.

### Healing and Repair

Healing and repair begin as soon as the inflammation has subsided and continue for several more days. There is an increase in capillary formation resulting in further development of granulation tissue. Collagen formation and fibroblastic activity continue, resulting in the formation of weak connective tissue. Clinically this stage can be recognized by a decrease in inflammation and pain.

*Treatment Objective:* During this stage of healing the main objective is to limit the formation of adhesions by utilizing a gentle, progressive approach to treatment.

### Remodelling

During the remodelling stage, which can be lengthy, the signs of inflammation are no longer present; the formation of collagen fibers becomes apparent. The connective tissue becomes stronger because of reorientation of collagen fibers in response to stresses. There is considerable overlap with the preceding stage and there may be recurrent episodes of dysfunction and pain.

*Treatment Objective:* The objective is full restoration of function, achieved by stretching and strengthening and by education of the patient.

## The Resistance-Pain Relationship in the Stages of Healing

According to Cyriax (1982) the relationship of resistance to passive movement and pain determines the stage of healing of a particular tissue and consequently the treatment approach that should be used. If, on the performance of passive movements, pain is experienced before resistance is felt the condition is in the **acute** (inflammatory) stage and treatment by movement should be of a very gentle nature, if at all.

When pain and resistance occur at the same time during the performance of passive movements the condition is in the **subacute** stage (healing and repair) and treatment by movement may proceed with caution.

Resistance appearing before pain during movement indicates that the condition is in the **chronic** stage (remodelling) and treatment approaches may be much more vigorous.

The treatment approaches used in each stage are determined by this relationship of resistance to pain.

## CARE OF THE PATIENT

Physical therapists spend a great deal of time with their patients on a one-to-one basis. Thus they are in a unique position in terms of patient care. In this section various aspects of patient care will be discussed, including: establishing a relationship and respect of privacy; comfortable positioning; clear instructions and demonstrations; care in handling; motivation and encouraging of independence; educating the patient; and some philosophical approaches to treatment.

## Establishing a Relationship

Patients do not visit hospitals or clinics from choice; they do so because they have a physical problem. They can, therefore, be apprehensive, easily intimidated, and very anxious. From the patient's point of view the most important time spent in contact with the physical therapist will occur in the first few minutes. The caring physical therapist will understand this and act accordingly.

Physical therapists, like other members of the health care team, have their own professional jargon. This specialized language use is important for communication with other members of the medical professions. However, it is completely out of place when communicating with a patient who is a **person first**. In establishing a relationship with the patient the recognition of the fact that she or he is a *person* (not a case) is the primary principle in establishing a successful relationship.

What does this mean? It means preparing a place in which the patient is going to be treated with privacy, greeting the patient in a warm and caring way by introducing oneself and enquiring about her or him, escorting the patient to the treatment area, and ensuring that she or he is comfortably situated and appropriately draped. In this way we have demonstrated that the patient is important.

The next step is to discuss, in **layman** terms, the patient's problem and the approach to treatment. It is important to allow time for the patient to ask questions and to make sure that she or he has fully understood the answers. Although this approach may seem time-consuming it will pay dividends in future therapist-patient contacts.

## Instructions and Demonstrations

It is important to ensure that clear instructions regarding the performance of movements are given, in layman terms, to the patient and that they are understood. Proper use of the voice with clear enunciation is of paramount importance. This communication process may be facilitated by usage of mirror image demonstrations by the therapist of the movements to be performed and then asking the patient to repeat them.

## Handling the Patient

At this stage in the care of the patient it may be assumed that she or he is comfortably situated in privacy and has confidence in the therapist. The laying on of hands is the next process. **However, it is very important that the therapist request permission to place his/her hands on the patient before doing so**. The therapist should be positioned relative to the patient so that the principles of good biomechanics are applied to both. The next step is to place the hands **gently** on the patient in such a way that the patient can become familiar with the therapist's touch and the therapist can become familiar with the state of the soft tissues requiring treatment. Increasing pressure and depth can be applied through the therapist's fingers as the patient's responses are monitored. The golden rule here is: **if you are going to err, do so gently**.

## Motivating and Educating the Patient Toward Independence

Too often patients bring their problems to the physical therapy department, dump them there for the physical therapist to do something with, and then take them home only to return to repeat the process a day or so later. **Passive therapy has its limitations**. Unless the patient is motivated to carry on at home with what has been taught by the therapist, a state of dependency is being encouraged. It follows then that after each treatment, involving **activity under instruction** on behalf of the patient, the patient should be asked to demonstrate to the therapist what she or he has been doing at home during the interim period.

## Treatment Approaches

It is vital to set short- and long-term objectives when treating a patient, based upon clinical findings. **Decreasing pain** is usually **the** short-term objective; during this period the patient is carefully monitored for exacerbation of pain. This initial goal is followed by associated, but longer-term, objectives related to restoring range of motion, muscle extensibility, strength, and normal function.

Treatment approaches are determined by the clinical features presented by the patient and by **individual characteristics and background medical knowledge of the patient**. Each patient is different and this fact must be considered when planning a treatment program; what will be successful in one patient may not be in another. There are numerous skillful treatment approaches available in the therapist's treatment bag. Often the therapist's experience and familiarity with a particular approach will determine the treatment to be used. There are, however, some basic rules which should be implemented.

It has already been mentioned that a comfortably situated and relaxed patient is essential to starting the treatment, and that attention to body biomechanics and gentle laying on of hands is of paramount importance.

A proximal to distal approach when treating hypomobility, muscle weakness, or both will ensure motion and stability throughout the kinetic chain. The performance of manual skills relating to joint hypomobility involves the application of firm but gentle grips; in both the mobilizing and stabilizing hands, the grips enhance the performance. Muscle weakness, which is treated initially by manual means, involves appropriate contact of the hands, clear instruction and demonstration, and careful application of resistance, as used in proprioceptive neuromuscular facilitation (PNF). This therapy has proved to be most beneficial.

## SUMMARY

This introductory chapter provided an overview of different aspects of musculoskeletal disorders. Initially the disorders were classified and then followed by common clinical findings. The stages of healing and their relationship to treatment objectives were briefly discussed. Next, various aspects of patient care were noted, such as establishing a relationship, giving clear instructions and demonstrations, and motivating and educating the patient toward independence. Finally, treatment objectives and principles of treatment were discussed.

CHAPTER 2

• • • • • • • •

# The Cervical Spine

The cervical spine extends from the occiput to the first thoracic verte-bra. The fact that the cervical spine is the most mobile part of the spinal column makes it vulnerable to injury and to degenerative changes.

## PERTINENT ANATOMICAL ASPECTS

The cervical spine is composed of seven vertebrae and their associ-ated soft tissue structures. It is divided into an upper and a lower cervical spine. The occiput and the first two vertebrae, the atlas and the axis, form the upper cervical spine and the third to seventh vertebrae form the lower cervical spine. The upper cervical spine is much more mobile than the lower cervical spine which has only small movements between one vertebra and the next. However, the cumulative movement in the lower cervical spine provides a good functional range of movement.

The main functions of the cervical spine are to support the head in space, facilitate its movements, and provide a route by which the brain is supplied by blood, and elements of the central nervous sys-tem gain access to the brain.

Certain structures of the cervical spine are more susceptible than others to adverse stresses and it therefore seems appropriate to review the pertinent anatomy of these structures before consid-ering the pathology associated with disorders of the cervical spine.

## The Functional Unit

The functional unit of the cervical spine consists of two vertebrae with an intervertebral disc (the intervertebral joint), an interverte-bral foramen (IVF), and two zygapophyseal joints and associated ligaments (Figure 2–1). Thus there is a three-joint complex. In addi-tion the joints of von Luschka can be identified on the posterolater-al aspects of the intervertebral joint.

### The Intervertebral Disc

Many spinal problems are caused by changes that occur in the intervertebral disc as a result of abnormal forces acting upon it. The changes may occur suddenly, as in traumatic incidents, or be insidious in onset, as in degeneration. Knowledge of the structure, function, and changes which can occur within a disc is necessary in order to understand what happens to the normal mechanics in disc problems (derangement syndromes).

**Structure.** Essentially the disc consists of two parts: a central nucleus pulposus and a peripheral annulus fibrosus (Figure 2–2). The nucleus is in contact with the cartilaginous vertebral end plate which contains numerous microscopic pores. These pores provide continuity between the nucleus and the spongy bone beneath the vertebral end plate (Kapandji, 1974).

**Nucleus Pulposus.** The nucleus is a transparent jelly containing 88 per cent water. There is a ground substance composed of proteogly-cans and water. The nucleus pulposus is roughly spherical in shape.

**Annulus Fibrosus.** This is made up of concentric rings of collagen fibers embracing the nucleus. The fibers of each ring, apart from the outermost one, run diagonally, each one in the opposite direc-tion to its neighbor. The obliquity increases the nearer the rings are to the nucleus, such that the fibers on the innermost ring are almost horizontal. The nucleus is thus embraced under pressure by the annulus fibrosus and is itself under tension.

**Nuclear Imbibition.** As stated previously the nucleus lies in contact with the vertebral end plates situated on the superior and inferior

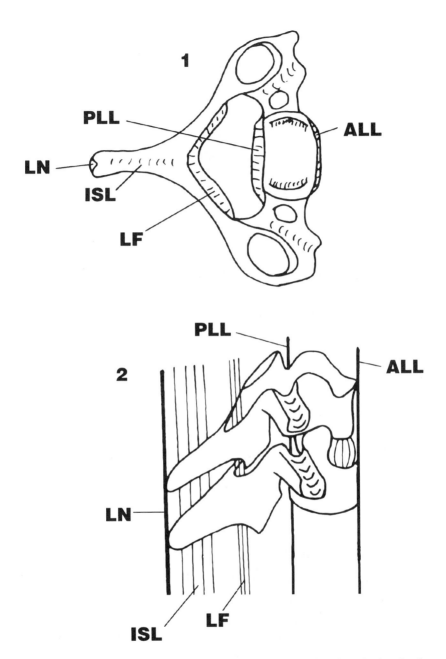

**Figure 2–1.** Ligamentous structures of the cervical spine. Anterior longitudinal ligament (ALL), posterior longitudinal ligament (PLL), ligamentum nuchae (LN), interspinous ligament (ISL), ligamentum flavum (LF). (1) Relationship to the cervical vertebra (adapted from Warwick & Williams, 1973). (2) Relationship to the functional unit (adapted from Foreman & Croft, 1988).

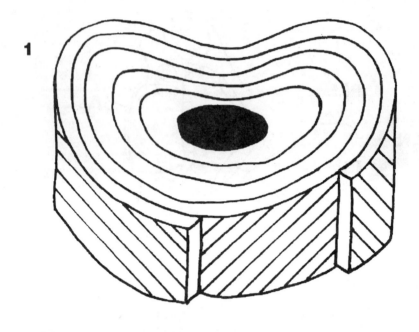

**1**

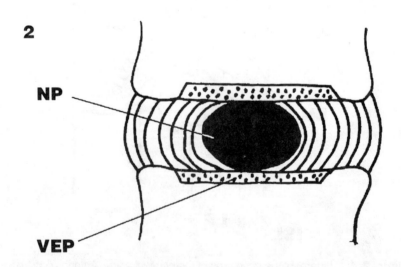

**2**

NP

VEP

**Figure 2–2.** The intervertebral disc: (1) central nucleus surrounded by the annulus fibrosus (adapted from Vernon-Roberts, 1987); and (2) relationship of the nucleus pulposus (NP) to the vertebral end plate (VEP) (adapted from Macnab, 1977).

surfaces of the vertebral body. The numerous tiny pores found in the end plates enable water to escape through these pores into the vertebral body when the nucleus is compressed. This loss of water from the discs amounts to a cumulative loss of height at the end of the day of approximately 2 cm. With assumption of the lying position during the night and a subsequent loss of compressive forces the disc regains its normal thickness as the water content returns. Clinically, most disc syndromes develop in the first few hours after waking when the nucleus has regained the normal fluid state. It appears that the spinal column is more vulnerable at this time, because of the increased flexibility.

With aging the disc is not able to readily absorb water through the process of imbibition because the degeneration which occurs blocks or destroys the tiny pores in the vertebral end plates. This fact explains the loss of flexibility and height in later years.

**Functions of the Disc.** These are as follows:

1. The nucleus pulposus acts as a shock absorber and distributor of mechanical stresses.
2. The disc facilitates smooth intervertebral movement; the nucleus acts as a fulcrum.
3. The annulus fibrosus acts as a check ligament for excessive movement.
4. The disc contributes to human height.
5. The disc is partly responsible for the normal curvature of the spinal column.
6. The nucleus plays a significant role in the exchange of nutrients and fluids between vertebra and disc.

**Nuclear Response to Spinal Movements.** According to Kapandji (1974) the nucleus responds to the different movements of the spine as follows:

- To flexion: The nucleus pulposus moves in a posterior direction.
- To extension: There is nuclear movement in an anterior direction.
- To lateral flexion: The nucleus will move to the side opposite to that to which the spine is flexing.

**Damage to the Annulus Fibrosus.** With an intact annulus the nucleus exerts equal pressure circumferentially. However, if the annular rings develop cracks nuclear material will tend to build up through the damaged annular rings, and bulging occurs. This bulging can cause pain as a result of pressure on pain sensitive structures such as the periphery of the annulus fibrosus and the posterior longitudinal ligament. There may also be interference with the normal mechanics of the disc, resulting in restriction of spinal movement. If the annulus breaks down completely the nuclear material will ooze out, resulting in a herniation of the nuclear material. Most disc syndromes are caused by bulging of nuclear material which is still contained by a weakened annulus. It is important to remember that because of the high water content of the nucleus the bulge is a "mobile" structure reducible by treatment approaches. Deviations in normal posture of the cervical and lumbar spines are frequently caused by a fluid buildup brought about by nuclear bulging, for example, posterior bulging causes kyphosis, lateral bulging causes scoliosis. Movements in a direction which would cause the vertebrae to "close the gap," thus restoring the fluid nucleus to its normal position, are used in treatment approaches; for example, extension would be used with a posterior protrusion because extension moves the fluid nucleus anteriorly towards its normal central location.

### The Intervertebral Foramen

The intervertebral foramen (IVF) has great clinical significance, particularly in the cervical spine, where it is more a tunnel than an opening. In order to better understand how the sensitive structures in the IVF become vulnerable to irritation or compression it is pertinent to review some of the anatomical aspects relating to this aperture.

The uncovertebral joints (joints of von Luschka), situated on the posterolateral rim of the vertebral body, form the anteromedial boundary of the foramen. The posterolateral boundary is formed by the zygapophyseal joints (facet joints).

The cross sectional area occupied by the nerve and dural sleeve makes up about one third to one half of the total area within the foramen. The remainder of the space is taken up by connective and areolar tissue, branches of the spinal artery, veins, lymphatic vessels, and filaments of the sinuvertebral nerve.

Under normal circumstances there is ample room within the intervertebral foramen for the nerve root. Irritation of the nerve root can however develop when the transverse diameter of the foramen is reduced by problems arising from the disc, the facet joint, or the uncovertebral joint, any one of which is capable of producing a space-occupying lesion.

Sudden trauma can cause disc lesions that result in the invasion of disc material into the foramen at a point lateral to the joints of von Luschka. Similarly the capsule of the facet joint can become swollen, thus taking up space posterolaterally. The nerve root itself can be subjected to a traction injury with resultant inflammation.

With the onset of degenerative changes osteophyte formation on the facet joints and joints of von Luschka gradually invades the foramen. The nerve root is capable of adjusting to a slow, gradual pressure, but eventually, continued invasion of the osteophytes will reduce the space to such an extent that painful symptoms develop. This is part of the explanation for the development of nerve root signs in the condition known as cervical spondylosis, a disorder that will be discussed later.

## Vertebral Arteries

The two vertebral arteries arise from the subclavian arteries and each ascends the cervical spine through the respective transverse foramina of the first six cervical vertebrae (Figure 2–3). On emerging from the transverse foramina of the first vertebra the two arteries pierce the posterior atlanto-occipital membrane and unite to form the basilar artery, which supplies the brain stem. The vertebral arteries are vulnerable to traction and compression forces on their passage through the transverse foramina. Cervical rotation will compromise the vertebral artery at the second cervical level; rotation to the right will compromise the left vertebral artery. Combined cervical rotation and extension can produce occlusion (Grant, 1988).

## Innervation of the Cervical Spine

The soft tissue structures of the cervical spine are innervated by branches from the anterior and posterior primary rami and the sinuvertebral nerve (Figure 2–4). Those structures anterior to the IVF are innervated by branches from the anterior primary ramus, and structures posterior to the IVF are innervated by branches from the posterior primary ramus. The sinuvertebral nerve innervates the

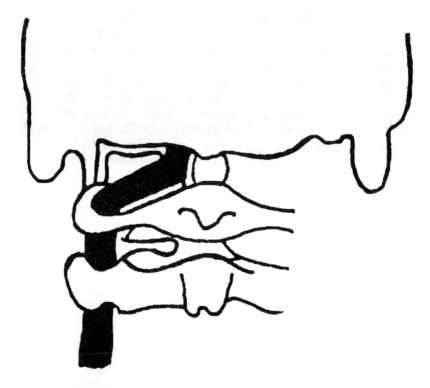

**Figure 2–3.** The left side of the upper cervical vertebrae and the left vertebral artery (adapted from Grieve, 1981).

periphery of the intervertebral disc, the dura mater, and the posterior longitudinal ligament.

## PAIN

Wyke (1987) has described pain as an abnormal affective state which differs from other affective states such as sadness or joy in that it is experienced in a particular part of the body. In the musculoskeletal system we are made aware of pain by virtue of the stimulation of the free nerve endings of the nociceptor system. These free nerve endings are found in the soft tissue structures of the musculoskeletal system, for instance in skin, muscle, tendon, or capsule of a joint. Under normal circumstances we are unaware of the activity of the nociceptor system until the soft tissues are sub-

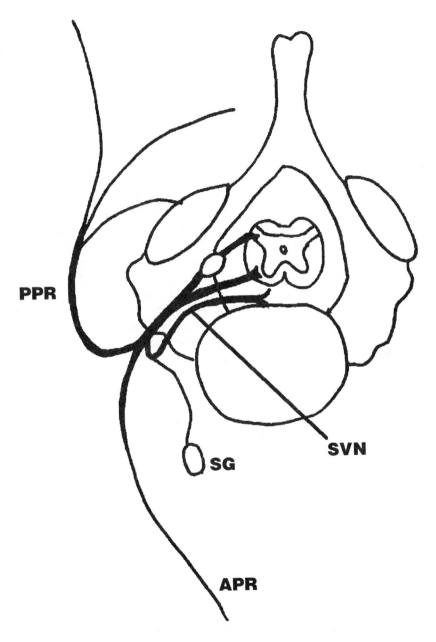

**Figure 2–4.** Innervation of the cervical spine. Posterior primary ramus (PPR), anterior primary ramus (APR), spinal ganglion (SG), and sinuvertebral nerve (SVN) (adapted from Cailliet, 1988).

jected to stress or trauma. When this happens there is an enhancement of the afferent activity of the nociceptor system resulting in pain. The system is particularly sensitive to mechanical **deformation of tissues**, and to **chemical irritation** caused, for instance, by an inflammatory reaction triggered by trauma. When caused by the former the pain is usually intermittent, unless the mechanical deformation is sustained. Pain attributable to chemical irritation is usually constant.

## Local and Referred Pain

Any structure that contains the free nerve endings described above can give rise to pain. Pain can manifest itself **locally**, when it is experienced by the patient at the site of the causative factor, for instance pain from a bruise caused by a blow on the arm. **Referred pain** is pain perceived by the patient to be in a location at a distance from the structure at fault. Pain from a source in the cervical spine can be experienced, for example in the anterior chest wall, the upper posterior thoracic region, the shoulder girdle, and the upper extremity; it is a common phenomenon in patients with conditions arising from the cervical spine. Referred pain can be divided into the following categories:

- *Nerve root pain* has been described as a lancinating or shooting type of pain with clearly defined borders; it is usually accompanied by distal paresthesia such as "pins and needles."
- *Somatic referred pain*, which is referred from **structures within the musculoskeletal system other than the nerve root**, has been described as a deep, boring ache that is diffuse in nature.
- *Visceral referred pain* arises from a disorder of an internal organ, such as the heart, that refers pain down the left arm; this tends to be diffuse in nature and it can be confused with somatic referred pain. A means of differentiation is that nerve root and somatic referred pain can be increased or decreased with movement but visceral pain remains unchanged.

## Pain Sensitive Soft Tissue Structures in the Spine

The following structures are innervated and are therefore capable of giving rise to pain. They are listed in an anterior to posterior direction:

1. skin, subcutaneous tissues, and musculature
2. anterior longitudinal ligament
3. intervertebral disc (periphery of the annulus)
4. periosteum of the vertebra
5. posterior longitudinal ligament (PLL)
6. ligamentum flavum
7. anterior part of the dura mater
8. dural sleeve of the nerve root
9. capsule of the zygapophyseal joints
10. interspinous ligaments
11. ligamentum nuchae
12. posterior musculature

In addition to the above structures, Wyke (1987) has pointed out that walls of blood vessels such as intramuscular arteries, epidural and paravertebral veins are also innervated and must be considered as a source of pain.

Bogduk (1986) has reported on documented experiments where hypertonic saline solution was injected into cervical interspinous ligaments and muscles. Referred pain to the head was produced by stimulation of upper cervical levels; stimulation of lower levels produced pain in the chest wall, shoulder girdle, and upper limb. He also noted that pressure on the PLL produces pain in the anterior chest.

## Stimulation of Different Parts of the Disc

The early work of Cloward (1959) on stimulating the different parts of the discs and noting where the subjects experienced pain provided us with much valuable information. He noted the following results of stimulation.

- Stimulation of the C3-C4 disc referred pain to the level of C7 spinous process.
- Stimulation of the C4-C5 disc referred pain to the superior angle of the scapula.
- Stimulation of the C5-C6 disc referred pain to the center of the vertebral border of the scapula.
- Stimulation of the C6-C7 disc referred pain to the inferior angle of the scapula.

*Note:* It is obvious from the above brief discussion of pain that it becomes increasingly difficult to categorically state that the pain is caused by this structure or that. The segmental theory (Cyriax, 1982), now discounted by some authors, has helped to explain some aspects of referred pain and continues to be a useful starting point in the assessment process. However, there is much more to learn about this phenomenon.

## WHIPLASH INJURY

Essentially whiplash is a soft tissue injury of the cervical spine.

## Mechanism of Injury

Whiplash commonly arises as a result of a rear end motor vehicle accident in which a stationary car is struck from behind by another vehicle that has failed to stop. The term "whiplash" describes the movement of the head and neck of the driver in the car that sustained the impact (Figure 2–5). Following the impact, the patient's trunk and the driver's seat move forward with the car (hence the term "acceleration injury"), but the head, which is unsupported, is thrown into hyperextension, subjecting the anterior cervical musculature to severe stretch. In response to the stretch the cervical musculature contracts and the head is brought forward into flexion. Also, as the car stops moving forward so does the patient's trunk, but the head continues to move forward. The range of extension is greater than that of flexion; the former is limited by the occiput striking the posterior chest wall and the latter is limited by the chin striking the sternum. Because the movement of the head simulates that of the lash of a whip the term "whiplash" is used to describe the injury. It would be more appropriate to describe it as a musculoligamentous strain or sprain of the cervical spine (Hirsch, Hirsch, Hiramoto, & Weiss, 1988). In addition to the above description of a whiplash injury there is the front-end impact where the driver of a car drives into a stationary vehicle. Under these circumstances the head first goes into flexion before recoiling into extension. This type of whiplash is also referred to as a "deceleration injury." It was hoped that the introduction of head rests would eliminate whiplash injuries; unfortunately, this has proved not to be so. Even with the use of the head rest severe injuries still occur because the body can move upwards beyond the support of the head rest.

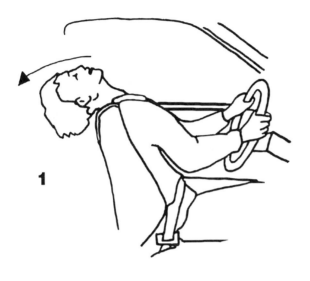

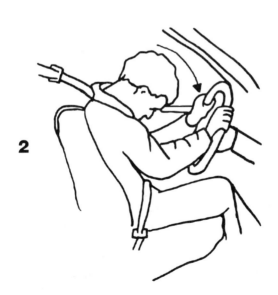

**Figure 2–5.** Mechanism of the whiplash injury: (1) the head and neck go into hyperextension during front end impact followed by (2) flexion of the head and neck.

## Pathology

Bogduk (1986) has identified the following structures as being sub-jected to strain or compression during the extension phase, then the flexion phase, of whiplash.

- Extension phase: prevertebral muscles, anterior longitudinal ligament, intervertebral discs, esophagus, odontoid process, zygapophyseal joints, spinous processes, temporomandibular joints, frontal and temporal lobes in the cranial fossae
- Flexion phase: vertebral bodies, intervertebral discs, inter-spinous ligament, zygapophyseal joints, ligamentum nuchae, posterior neck muscles

In addition to the above injury sites, nerve root compression and breast trauma (the latter as a result of wearing the diagonal strap of a seat belt) have also been identified (Foreman & Croft, 1988). Downs and Twomey (1979) mention the vertebral artery and the sympathetic chain as vulnerable structures in the whiplash injury.

The extent to which the above structures will be damaged is determined by the following factors:

- the force of the impact;
- whether or not the patient saw the offending vehicle coming and was able to brace against the impact;
- the position of the patient's neck at the time of the impact; if the patient's neck is rotated, the range of extension will be decreased (Macnab, 1971) and damage to the anterior struc-tures will be reduced.

## Clinical Features

It is not uncommon for symptoms to be delayed for periods of sev-eral hours or days (Hirsch et al. 1988). Once they become estab-lished, all or some of the following clinical features may be present:

- sore, aching neck and shoulder
- swelling of soft structures of the anterior cervical spine
- muscle spasm
- nausea and vomiting
- pain in the interscapular region and arm pain (the latter may be nerve root pain or somatic referred pain)

- headache caused by C1-C3 nerve root involvement (Bogduk, 1986)
- paresthesia and numbness
- temporomandibular joint problems as a result of the head being thrown into hyperextension and the mandible dropping
- dizziness, tinnitus, nystagmus, and blurring of vision, all of which are indicative of involvement of the vertebral artery and sympathetic chain
- muscle weakness and muscle tenderness in related myotomes
- dysphagia—caused by bleeding in the retropharyngeal space
- elevation of the scapula on the affected side—to ease the tension on the nerve roots or tight musculature
- hyperesthesia as reported by Reichl and Allen (1987)
- deafness
- low back pain which initially may be masked by more severe symptoms.

In terms of prognosis, Foreman and Croft (1988) developed a numerical scale that enabled them to objectively classify whiplash injuries. Three major injury categories (MIC) were established and assigned a numerical value; for example, MIC 1 was assigned 10 points. Next, significant modifiers to prognosis were identified and graded on a point system; for example, kyphotic curve was assigned 15 points and preexisting degeneration was assigned 10 points. The points for the significant modifiers were added to the points assigned to the patient's MIC category; five prognosis groups were established with prognosis group five carrying the most points and hence the worst prognosis.

## Treatment Guidelines

The treatment of the whiplash patient is determined by the severity of the injury. The single most important component is the supportive role of the therapist in trying to relate symptomatology (often unexpected) to pathology. The following protocol is for a severe whiplash injury; although this has been divided into stages, inevitably there will be overlap from one stage to the next.

### Acute Stage

The acute stage treatment consists of:

- rest in bed with a soft collar;
- ice application if tolerated;

- encouragement in relaxation of neck musculature and gentle active movements in a pain-free range;
- analgesics and muscle relaxants.

### Subacute Stage

The subacute stage treatment protocol is:

- encouragement to discard the collar except at night;
- transcutaneous electrical nerve stimulation (TENS);
- isometric exercises;
- soft tissue mobilization in the form of relaxation and gentle oscillatory movements, particularly in the suboccipital region;
- postural correction with chin retraction;
- active exercises for cervical spine and upper extremity;
- manual traction;
- education in care of the neck.

### Chronic Stage

In the chronic stage the treatment is:

- home traction;
- myofascial release techniques.

*Note:* The patient with the whiplash injury has been much maligned in the past, largely because of ignorance on the part of the health care professional. Patients with a severe whiplash injury may be permanently disabled in one way or another. As with all patients, they warrant as much help and consideration as physical therapists can provide.

## CERVICAL SPONDYLOSIS

Cervical spondylosis is a degenerative condition present in varying degrees in most people beyond the age of 40 years. Macnab (1975) explains how spondylosis initially affects the cervical discs then progresses to involve the vertebral bodies, zygapophyseal joints, the joints of von Luschka, and the ligamentous structures (Figure 2–6). The entire cervical spine can be affected by the degenerative process; C5-C6 level is most frequently involved and the C6-C7 level is the next most frequently involved (Lestini & Wiesel, 1989).

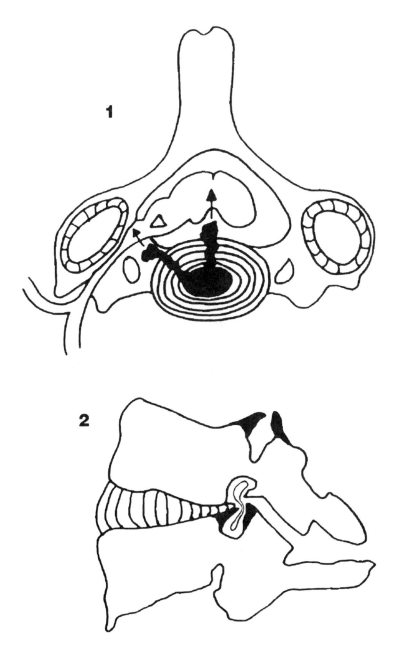

**Figure 2–6.** Stages of cervical spondylosis: (1) disc degeneration with nuclear displacement; and (2) osteophytic formation on the vertebral bodies and the zygapophyseal joint (adapted from Kapandji, 1974).

## Pathology

The degeneration begins in the nucleus pulposus as a result of loss of hydration; consequently the ability of the disc to act as a shock absorber is diminished. This creates more stress on the annulus fibrosus resulting in tears in the annulus and the predisposition to herniation of the disc. Excessive forces are also placed on the associated structures such as the facet joints, joints of von Luschka, and ligaments (Shelokov, 1991). The effect of this degenerative process and loss of disc height creates an unstable situation in the spine; it is during this stage that the spine is apt to be injured (Macnab, 1975). This unstable situation is offset eventually by the formation of osteophytes on the superior and inferior surfaces of the vertebral bodies, the joints of von Luschka and the facet joints due to hypertrophy and calcification which increase stability but cause a loss of motion.

Macnab (1975) has shown that loss of height posteriorly in the intervertebral joint can continue only to the point where the component parts of the joints of von Luschka come into contact; further loss of disc height will result in loss of height in the **anterior** aspect of the intervertebral joint with consequent flexion of the cervical spine.

It is important to remember that even in the presence of notable pathological changes, as evidenced by X-ray, cervical spondylosis is often asymptomatic. However, symptoms can arise during the **unstable stage** as a result of superimposed trauma or postural strain affecting the ligamentous structures and the capsules of the zygapophyseal joints.

In the **later stages of degeneration** nerve root pain can develop as a result of compression of the nerve root by the disc material. If the degeneration affects the size of the spinal canal a cervical myelopathy can result.

## Clinical Features

The clinical features of cervical spondylosis will be described in terms of the unstable stage and the later stages of the degenerative process.

### Unstable Stage

In the unstable stage we find:

- sore aching neck with limitation of movement;
- muscle spasm;

- headaches in the suboccipital region;
- muscles of the shoulder girdle and scapula may be sore;
- somatic referred pain into one or both upper limbs may be present;
- articular signs relating to disc protrusion (Cyriax, 1971).

### Later Stages of the Degenerative Process

In the later stages these are the clinical features:

- nerve root pain commonly from C6 or C7 nerve roots (Cyriax, 1982; Macnab, 1975);
- associated shooting, stabbing pain, paresthesia, muscle tenderness and weakness, diminished reflexes, and loss of sensation arising from involvement of C6 or C7 nerve roots;
- vertebral artery symptoms caused by encroachment of osteophytes into the transverse foramina (Pryse-Phillips & Murray, 1982);
- signs of upper motor neuron disease, for example, clumsy gait caused by compression of the spinal cord (Shelokov, 1991).

## Treatment Guidelines

Treatment guidelines are presented first for the unstable stage and then for the later stages of the degenerative process.

### Unstable Stage

Pain occurs as a result of synovitis of the capsule of the zygapophyseal joint, ligamentous sprain, and muscle strain.

The instability is related to interference in the normal mechanics of the functional unit as a result of disc degeneration plus a loss of integrity of the ligamentous structures. The following procedures may be tried:

- rest in a soft collar may be necessary;
- avoidance of irritating repetitive movements of the neck or upper limb and of prolonged postures
- hot packs;
- postural correction and education in the care of the cervical spine;
- isometric exercises.

When articular signs are evident in the early stages Cyriax (1971, 1984) advocates manipulative reduction by utilizing strong manual traction and circumduction or strong manual traction with rotation.

### Later Stages of the Degenerative Process

If cord signs or the vertebral artery syndrome (dizziness, double vision, drop attacks, interference with speech, and difficulty in swallowing) are present and the results of tests indicate that the problem is osteophytic encroachment, the only recourse is surgical intervention.

Cyriax (1971) believed that the term cervical spondylosis should be used only when osteophyte compression of the cord or nerve roots is present and that until this happens the process is one of natural degeneration that is ultimately present in everyone, and is, in most cases, symptom free. Bland (1987) prefers to use the term cervical osteoarthritis to describe all joint involvement in the cervical spine, including all secondary manifestations in vertebrae, tendons, ligaments, capsules, muscles, and hyaline cartilage.

Bland refuses to make the assumption that the disorder begins in the intervertebral disc. He agrees with Cyriax that in many instances the patient is asymptomatic.

## CERVICAL DISC LESIONS

Lesions of the cervical disc are fairly common disorders. Bulging of the disc can affect the nerve root **below the level of the affected disc,** for example, the disc at C5-C6 level will impinge upon the C6 nerve root. The cervical disc at C6-C7 level resulting in a C7 nerve root problem, is the most frequent finding in cervical disc disorders (Cyriax, 1982). Lestini and Wiesel (1989) believe the C5 and C6 nerve roots are those most often involved.

## Etiology

The causes of cervical disc lesions commonly evolve from the following events:

- trauma is a likely cause, particularly in the presence of existing degeneration of the cervical spine;

- a patient may wake up with the problem, having had the head in a poor postural position for an extended period of time, or it may develop shortly after waking;
- a sudden movement can be a precipitating factor.

## Clinical Features

General signs and symptoms are presented first, followed by those of the full root cervical syndromes.

### General Signs and Symptoms

The signs and symptoms are:

- some movements are painful and restricted, others are not;
- scapular pain is very common;
- shoulder and upper arm pain is usually present;
- paresthesia (pins and needles) in the fingers may be a complaint;
- diminished reflexes are often found;
- muscle weakness may be present.

### Full Root Cervical Syndromes

Full root syndromes have been described in detail by Cyriax (1982) and are listed below. The pain experienced by the patient will be felt in the appropriate dermatome (Figures 2–7 and 2–8).

C5 nerve root
- Pain extends from the scapular region, and down the front of the arm and forearm to the radial hand, stopping at the base of the thumb.
- Paresthesia is not present.
- Muscle weakness is evident in the C5 myotome—deltoid, spinati, biceps.
- Biceps and brachioradialis reflex responses are sluggish.

C6 nerve root
- Pain follows a pattern in the arm and forearm similar to that of the C5 nerve root since there is considerable overlap between these two dermatomes.

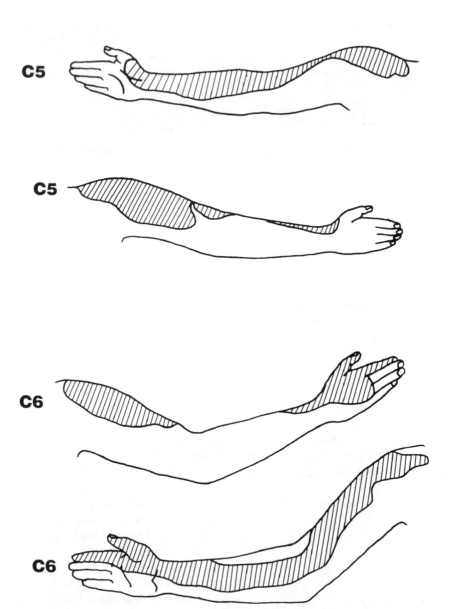

C5

C5

C6

C6

**Figure 2–7.** Cervical dermatomes C5-C6.

34

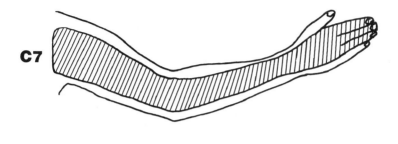

C7

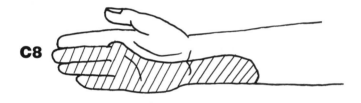

C8

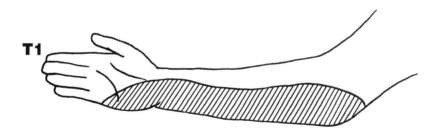

T1

**Figure 2–8.** Cervical dermatomes C7-C8 and the first thoracic dermatome T1.

- Paresthesia in the form of pins and needles is felt in the thumb and index finger.
- There is weakness of brachialis, biceps, and brachioradialis.
- The biceps jerk may be absent or sluggish.

C7 nerve root
- Pain extends from the scapular area, down the back of the arm and outer forearm to the index, long, and ring fingers. There is usually paresthesia (pins and needles) in the first three fingers also.
- Weakness of the triceps is the outstanding weakness; the biceps reflex is usually normal.
- Weakness of the wrist flexors may be present.
- Numbness is felt on the dorsum of the long and index fingers.

C8 nerve root
- There is lower scapular pain that extends to the inner side (or back) of the arm and medial forearm.
- Pins and needles are present in 3rd, 4th, and 5th fingers (Figure 2–8).
- Flexor carpi ulnaris, adductor and extensor pollicis, and extensor digitorum communis are usually weak.
- There is numbness of the little finger.

### Differential Diagnosis

Cyriax (1982) has emphasized the importance of differential diagnosis; some of the conditions with which the different nerve root syndromes can be confused are identified below.

C5 nerve root
- Suprascapular nerve disorder
- Rupture of the spinati muscles
- Secondary malignant deposits in the scapula

C6 nerve root
- Tennis elbow
- Rupture of biceps
- Carpal tunnel syndrome
- Pressure on the lower trunk of the brachial plexus

C7 nerve root

- Carcinoma of the bronchus
- Tennis elbow or golfer's elbow

C8 nerve root

- Malignancy of the 7th cervical or 1st thoracic vertebrae resulting in extreme weakness. Malignancy is usually identifiable by a double root weakness C7 + 8 or C8 + T1. In non-malignant circumstances single nerve roots are involved in disc problems affecting the cervical spine.
- Angina
- Cervical rib causing weakness in T1 myotome

## Treatment

Cyriax, McKenzie, and Maitland all offer useful treatment approaches for cervical disc lesions.

Cyriax (1984) advocates manipulation with strong traction, providing certain criteria are met, such as the absence of neurological deficits. Postural education is an important component and a collar is helpful in maintaining the reduction in unstable situations. Home traction may also be part of the treatment protocol. Exercises are not encouraged until the condition is stabilized (Cyriax, 1982).

McKenzie (1990) is concerned with determining which repetitive movement during his testing procedures relieves or centralizes the patient's pain and thus reduces the derangement. He then instructs the patient in the regular use of that movement over a period of 24 hours. The use of a lumbar roll in correction of posture in the sitting position and good positioning of the head and neck are emphasized (Figure 2–9). Once reduction is achieved the next step is to maintain the reduction. When the pain has been eliminated or extensively diminished for a period of 24 hours the reduction is considered to be stable and recovery of function can commence. Flexion exercises should be introduced as soon as possible, followed by movements in all directions. The patient is placed on a self-treatment approach (McKenzie, 1983).

Maitland (1986) uses cervical rotations towards the pain-free side and oscillatory pressures on the spinal process of the appropriate vertebra. Intermittent traction with the cervical spine in flexion has been found useful for patients with severe pain arising from disc disorders of the lower cervical spine.

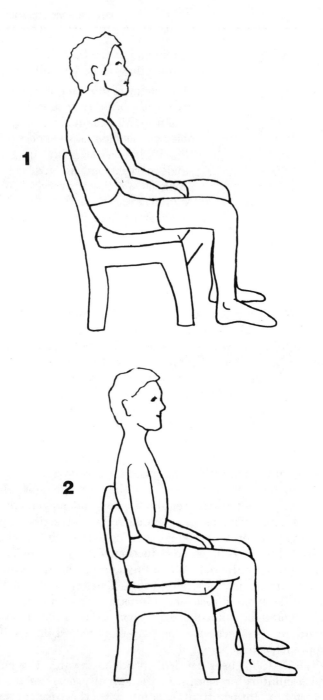

**Figure 2–9.** Sitting postures: (1) the slouch position; (2) the correct sitting position (adapted from McKenzie, 1990).

The use of a soft collar is helpful providing the patient does not become dependent.

## THORACIC OUTLET SYNDROME

Thoracic outlet syndrome is caused by compression of the neurovascular bundle or of any of its components, for example, the subclavian artery or vein, or of the roots of the brachial plexus. The cause of the compression is usually an abnormal bony structure (cervical rib) or an abnormality of soft tissue such as an anomaly of the scalene muscles. However, the condition can result from trauma to the cervical spine or the upper extremity. The three-minute elevation test described by Howell (1987), compresses all three components of the neurovascular bundle. Two different neurological patterns, one involving C5-C7 and the other involving C8-T1, have been identified; the latter is the most common pattern.

## Levels of Compression

For convenience the four regions where compression occurs can be described in relation to the clavicle (Figure 2–10).

### Above the Clavicle

1. at the lower part of the neck as a result of a cervical rib (extra rudimentary rib arising from the seventh cervical vertebra)
2. between scalenus anterior and scalenus medius (the scalenus anterior syndrome)

### At the Level of the Clavicle

3. between the clavicle and the first rib (the costoclavicular syndrome)

### Below the Clavicle

4. beneath pectoralis minor (the hyperabduction syndrome)

Bateman (1972) and Howell (1987) believe that the term thoracic inlet syndrome (TIS) is a more appropriate description since

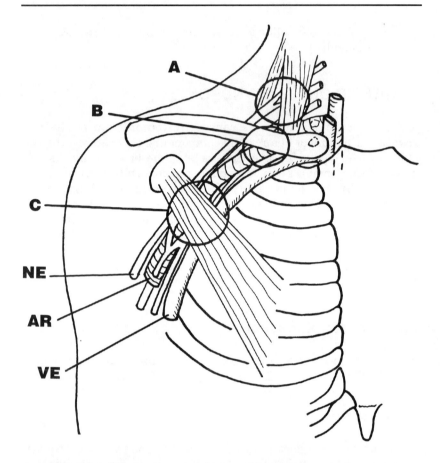

**Figure 2-10.** The thoracic outlet, areas of compression, and the neurovascular bundle. Scalenus anterior syndrome (A), costoclavicular syndrome (B), hyperabduction syndrome (C), nerve (N), artery (AR), and vein (VE).

the problem develops in the region of the entrance to the thoracic cage rather than the exit.

## Etiology

Generally, the compression arises as a result of a bony or soft tissue abnormality. Other than the cervical rib the following abnormalities can occur:

- abnormal insertion of the scalene muscles, spasm, or hypertrophy of these muscles;
- deformities of the clavicle as a result of malunion of fractures which result in a decrease in size of the costoclavicular space;
- tight pectoralis minor.

## Clinical Features

If the lower part of the plexus is compressed the patient's symptoms will be located in the medial part of the arm, forearm, and hand (almost certainly the latter). The lateral part of the arm, forearm, and hand is affected if the C5-C7 part of the plexus is involved.

The following symptoms relate to compression of the roots of the brachial plexus:

- pain;
- paresthesia;
- muscle weakness.

Symptoms associated with vascular involvement are:

- edema of the hand;
- a feeling of heaviness of the upper extremity;
- color changes in the hand similar to those found in Raynaud's disease.

### Differential Tests

The following tests assist the therapist in determining the level where the compression is taking place.

**Adson's Test for Scalenus Anterior.** The patient is asked to hyperextend the head and rotate it towards the affected side, while taking a deep breath. The head movement puts the scalenus anterior on full stretch; since this muscle is inserted into the first rib the subclavian artery is compressed between the first rib and the clavicle. Further compression is achieved by asking the patient to take in a deep breath which also elevates the first rib. The patient's pulse is monitored with the arm at the side. Decrease in pulse strength or its obliteration is a positive indicator.

**Costoclavicular Test.** People who carry pack bags on their backs, or who have an exaggerated military posture, may also exhibit a narrowing of the space between the clavicle and first rib. To test for this, the patient is asked to retract and depress the shoulder girdle with the arms relaxed by the sides. This maneuver narrows the space between the clavicle and the first rib even more, thus compromising the neurovascular bundle. Once again the pulse is monitored; reproduction of the patient's symptoms or a diminished or lost pulse is a positive result for the test.

**The Hyperabduction Test (Wright's Test).** The neurovascular bundle can become compressed between the costocoracoid membrane and the pectoralis minor. The symptoms can be reproduced by hyperabducting the arm, thus stretching the muscle and further compressing the sensitive structures beneath. If the pulse is monitored in the hyperabducted position it will be diminished sooner on the affected side and the uncomfortable symptoms will appear. However, loss of the pulse is not the significant sign since in many normals the pulse will disappear with the arm in this position. Bateman (1972) has indicated that pressure applied over the pectoralis minor just below the coracoid, with the patient in the sitting position, will also reproduce the painful symptoms. The person who habitually sleeps on the side with the abducted arm underneath the head often complains of TOS symptoms.

**The Three-Minute Elevation Test.** This test has been designed to detect TOS whatever the cause may be. It is a recent development compared with the other tests described and is increasing in popularity.

The patient is placed in the sitting position and is asked to abduct the shoulders to 90° with the elbows bent to 90° and the shoulders slightly braced. The patient is asked to repeatedly clench and open the fists slowly for three minutes. If the patient has TOS the symptoms will be reproduced during the test.

TOS can be confused with myofascial pain syndromes (Travell & Simons, 1983), with nerve root problems arising from the cervical spine, and with somatic referred pain caused by injured cervical spine structures. From the results of a study carried out by Carroll and Hurst (1982) it became clear that carpal tunnel syndrome with associated shoulder pain can also be easily confused with TOS.

## Treatment Guidelines

These essentially consist of a stretching, mobilizing, strengthning, and a postural program. Smith (1979) has described such a program that includes the following procedures:

- mobilization of the sternoclavicular and acromioclavicular joints and the first and second ribs to increase the costoclavicular space;
- stretching of the scalene and pectoral muscles to restore extensibility;
- correction of posture and strengthening of weakened muscles;
- correction of poor sleeping habits such as lying with the head on the hyperabducted arm.

*Note:* Howell (1987) presents a thorough evaluation of the patient with TOS; it includes a detailed postural examination, an evaluation of soft tissue restrictions, examination of muscles for myofascial trigger points, motion testing, provocative maneuvers, and sensory and sympathetic evaluation. The principle of treatment is similar to that described by Smith (1979) in that the focus is on postural correction and maintenance. A three phase treatment program is instituted:

- control of the patient's pain;
- correction of the musculoskeletal postural faults;
- inclusion of a postural maintenance program.

## ACUTE TORTICOLLIS

Acute torticollis is also referred to as wry neck, which infers a lateral flexion deformity or cervical scoliosis. It occurs in children or young adults and affects the segments between C2 and C7, most commonly C2-C3 (Grieve, 1981).

## Mechanism of Onset

A slight shift in nuclear material is a possible mechanism of onset.

## Clinical Features

The child or young adult may waken in the middle of the night complaining of pain on one side of the neck; alternatively the child may arise in the morning with a painful neck.

The head is held in slight forward flexion and lateral flexion away from the affected side.

The pain is usually localized on the convex side of the neck, but if the condition does not resolve it can spread to the scapular region and outer and posterior aspects of the arm (Grieve, 1981).

Lateral flexion to the affected side and extension are limited because of pain. Rotation to either side is painful, but the range is limited toward the affected side (Maitland, 1986).

## Treatment

If the condition is minor it can correct spontaneously (Corrigan & Maitland, 1983). If it persists, gentle rotations to the affected side (or the unaffected side if pain is exacerbated) are often effective; these are followed by traction in flexion for 15 minutes (Maitland, 1986).

An alternative approach is to apply a hot pack with the neck in a comfortable position and to encourage the patient to do gentle physiological rotations to the affected side if tolerated; if pain is exacerbated, gentle physiological rotations to the unaffected side should be initiated first.

## CERVICAL JOINT LOCK

Cervical joint lock syndrome shares certain similarities with the acute torticollis described previously and as a result may be confused with the latter.

## Mechanism of Onset

Cervical joint lock develops as the result of a sudden movement of the cervical spine (Sprague, 1983; and Maitland, 1986), with subsequent trapping of a meniscoid structure between the articular surfaces of the zygapophyseal joint (Grieve, 1981).

## Clinical Features

Following the precipitating movement the patient, usually a young adolescent, finds the head appears to be locked in a position of lateral flexion and rotation away from the affected side. There is a local focus of pain on the convex side of the neck, commonly at the level of C2-C3 (Grieve, 1981; Maitland, 1986).

Lateral flexion and rotation toward the painful side are limited as is extension.

There is restriction of passive intervertebral movement at the involved level.

## Treatment Guidelines

The following guidelines have met with success in the management of cervical joint lock:

- longitudinal oscillatory traction;
- physiological rotation to the unaffected then the affected side;
- manipulation.

## SUMMARY

The chapter began with a review of the pertinent anatomy related to the conditions under discussion. Because pain is an integral component of these conditions a brief review of this symptom in terms of local and referred pain and pain-sensitive structures in the cervical spine was also included. The first topic to be discussed was the Whiplash injury; there is much about this condition that is yet to be discovered and the patient suffering from this disorder is often maligned. The degenerative processes resulting in Spondylosis of the cervical spine were discussed next; a section on Cervical Disc Lesions followed. The Thoracic Outlet Syndrome continues to be something of an enigma and can be confused with other conditions with similar symptomatology; this too was noted in the chapter. Acute Torticollis was defined and discussed; distinction was made between it and Cervical Joint Lock.

CHAPTER 3

• • • • • • • •

# The Shoulder Complex

The shoulder complex of joints sustains more injuries than any other part of the upper extremity; it consists of the following:

- the scapulothoracic 'joint';
- the acromioclavicular joint;
- the sternoclavicular joint;
- the glenohumeral joint;
- the subdeltoid 'joint' (Kapandji, 1982).

## FUNCTIONAL ASPECTS

The function of these joints is to facilitate movement of the upper extremity in order to ensure appropriate placing of the hand for effective use. The joints are interdependent and move in concert with one another. Kapandji (1982) describes direct links among the first three joints listed above and direct links between the last two joints. It follows then that a problem with one of these joints could affect the function of the others.

Cailliet (1988) and Kaput (1987) both feel that the costosternal and costovertebral joints should be included when describing the shoulder complex. It is important to bear these joints in mind since they are not generally included in an assessment of the shoulder complex. The mobility of the upper thoracic spine should also be examined as hypomobility can affect shoulder position and function (Cailliet, 1966; Grieve, 1981).

**47**

## RELATIONSHIP OF THE CERVICAL
## SPINE TO SHOULDER PAIN

Wells (1982) pointed out that painful disorders of the glenohumeral joint frequently have their origin in the cervical spine. Maigne (1972) believes that **an examination of the cervical spine should be carried out whenever a painful shoulder exists**. Kessel (1982) has stated that in one fifth of patients with shoulder pain the pain is referred from the cervical spine. Indeed, eliminating the cervical spine as the cause of pain in the glenohumeral joint is an important preliminary step in problems involving the shoulder complex.

## PERTINENT ANATOMY

Common afflictions of the shoulder complex are those involving the soft tissue structures of the glenohumeral joint and particularly the muscles of the rotator cuff (Figure 3–1). The muscles, in conjunction with the subacromial bursa, cover the head of the humerus and include supraspinatus, infraspinatus, teres minor, and subscapularis. Their collective function is to retain the head of the humerus in the glenoid cavity. The long head of biceps (Figure 3–2) is closely associated with muscles of the rotator cuff and is sometimes regarded as the fifth rotator cuff muscle. The supraspinatus, anterior aspect of infraspinatus, and biceps tendon are the structures most prone to injury. Certainly these tendons are prone to overuse syndromes; the supraspinatus is particularly vulnerable. Injuries to these soft tissue structures will be discussed later in this chapter.

The humeral component of the glenohumeral joint is susceptible to injuries resulting in fractures; these are described in Chapter 11. Injuries to the acromioclavicular joint and its ligamentous structures occur fairly often in athletic activities and these will be discussed next.

## ACROMIOCLAVICULAR INJURIES

Problems involving the acromioclavicular (AC) joint are fairly common in athletes; these usually result in a partial or complete separation of the joint (Figure 3–3). Other problems of the joint can develop indirectly from overuse as a result of abnormal mobility elsewhere in the complex, for example, the scapulothoracic mechanism (Macnab & Hastings, 1968).

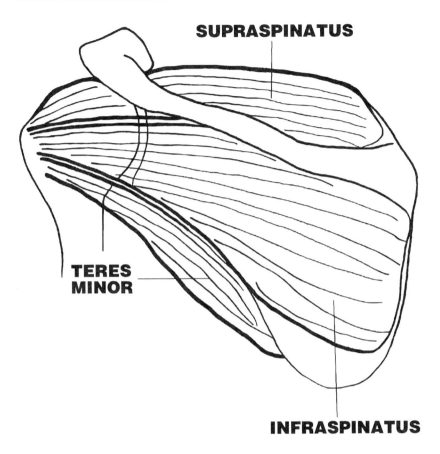

**Figure 3–1.** The three rotator cuff muscles arising from the posterior surface of the scapula (adapted from Netter, 1989).

## Mechanism of Injury

The most common mechanisms involve football or motor vehicle accidents (Stewart, 1985), in which the acromion, scapula and upper extremity are driven inferiorly and the supporting ligamentous structures are sprained or torn (R.J. Neviaser, 1987a).

## Classification and Treatment

There is some general agreement regarding the classification of injuries to the ligamentous structures of the AC joint, but unanim-

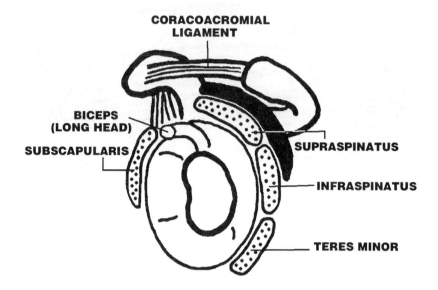

**Figure 3–2.** The lateral aspect of the glenohumeral joint with the humerus removed showing the subacromial space and the muscles of the rotator cuff (adapted from Netter, 1989).

ity does not exist in terms of treatment approaches. It is generally agreed that there are three grades of injury (R.J. Neviaser, 1987a). Reid (1992) describes six grades, the last three being extensions of Grade III.

### Grade I

A Grade I injury is a partial tear of the capsule and associated acromioclavicular ligament without displacement of the joint. Treatment consists of ice and analgesics employed initially with rest in a sling until the acute symptoms subside. Following the period of rest, strengthening exercises, stretching, and functional activities are added.

### Grade II

A Grade II injury involves a rupture of the acromioclavicular ligament with a partial tear of the coracoclavicular ligament producing a subluxation (R.J. Neviaser, 1987a). This type of injury can be treated conservatively with sling support, or it can be treated surgically.

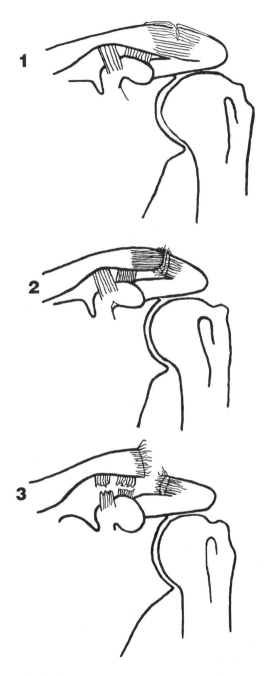

**Figure 3–3.**  Injuries to the acromioclavicular joint (1) grade one injury, (2) grade two injury, and (3) grade three injury (adapted from Neviaser, R.J. 1987a).

The latter approach is utilized for patients involved in contact sports, or for those patients involved in heavy manual labor. Surgery involves repair of the ligaments and the deltoid and trapezius muscles, if the latter are torn. A sling is worn until the ligaments are healed. Rehabilitation, as described for a Grade I injury, restores muscle strength and joint stability.

### Grade III

In Grade III injuries there is a complete rupture of the acromioclavicular and coracoclavicular ligaments with dislocation of the joint. This is the injury that is often described as joint "separation." The common surgical approach is to remove the lateral end of the clavicle and repair the ligaments. However, not all patients are treated surgically; some Grade III injuries respond just as well to reduction of the dislocation, followed by placing the arm in a broad arm sling during the painful period—about 2–3 weeks (Dias & Gregg, 1991; R.J. Neviaser, 1987a). Exercises are commenced as soon as the pain permits (Dias & Gregg, 1991).

*Note:* Studies indicate that patients undergoing early operative treatment and those treated conservatively present with similar results (Dias & Gregg, 1991; R.J. Neviaser, 1987a).

## THE IMPINGEMENT SYNDROME

The area in which impingement occurs is the subacromial space (Figure 3–4); it is bounded superiorly by the acromion and the coracoacromial ligament which form the coracoacromial arch, and inferiorly by the head of the humerus and its associated soft tissue structures, including the subacromial bursa.

## Predisposing Factors

A relatively avascular area has been identified in the tendon of supraspinatus just proximal to its insertion on the humerus. Rathbun and Macnab (1970) have shown that with the arm in the abducted position the blood vessels fill, but that there is a depletion of blood with the arm at the side. Lohr and Uhthoff (1990) have shown that the avascularity is greater on the articular side of the tendon of supraspinatus than on the bursal side. There is also an area of avascularity in the intracapsular portion of the long head of the biceps tendon (Fink & Welsh, 1990). These areas of avasculari-

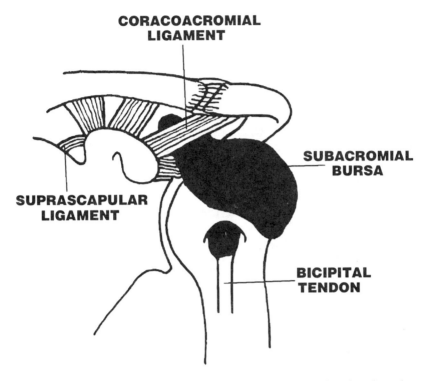

**CORACOACROMIAL LIGAMENT**

**SUBACROMIAL BURSA**

**SUPRASCAPULAR LIGAMENT**

**BICIPITAL TENDON**

**Figure 3–4.** Anterior aspect of the glenohumeral joint showing the relationship of the subacromial bursa to the coracoacromial ligament (adapted from Netter, 1989).

ty make the tendons susceptible to degenerative changes. Involvement of the bursa is usually a secondary manifestation. The normal gliding mechanism afforded by the bursa is lost as it becomes thickened and the impingement increases because of further loss of the confined space.

## Etiological Factors

Cailliet (1966) has shown that postural defects resulting in hypomobility can result in impingement. An excessive thoracic kyphosis as seen in the elderly, in the depressed individual, or in one who continually assumes a slumped posture at work, depresses the coracoacromial arch and leads to internally rotated shoulders. Both factors will cause impingement of the soft tissue structures surrounding the head of the humerus against the overlying arch. Round shoulders have the effect of depressing the glenoid cavity and the coracoacromial arch causing impingement to occur early in the range.

The impingement syndrome has also been described as an overuse syndrome: individuals who are most at risk are those who, during occupational or sporting activities, use their arms above the horizontal in the forward flexed position (Hawkins & Abrams, 1987; Neviaser & Neviaser, 1990). In forward flexion of the arm, which has been described by Neer (1972) as the "functional arc of elevation," the greater tuberosity of the humerus and its associated soft tissue structures may impinge against the anterior one third of the acromion. If internal rotation is added in the forward flexed position, impingement will occur against the coracoacromial ligament. The structures most commonly implicated are the supraspinatus tendon and the long head of biceps. T.J. Neviaser (1987a) has stated that clinical differentiation between these two structures is not easy. The subdeltoid bursa becomes involved as a secondary manifestation.

Repeated elevation through abduction without the accompanying external rotation will also cause the impingement syndrome.

## Pathology

Neer and Welsh (1977) and Neer (1983) have identified three stages of the impingement syndrome.

1. *Edema and Hemorrhage.* This stage corresponds to a tendinitis of the involved tendon(s); most commonly affected is supraspinatus, then the long head of biceps. Infraspinatus is also frequently involved.
2. *Thickening and Fibrosis of the Involved Tendon(s) and Bursa.*
3. *Rotator Cuff Tears, Biceps Rupture, and Bony Changes.* The latter develop on the head of the humerus, the acromioclavicular joint, and the coracoacromial ligament.

## Clinical Features

### Stage One (Tendinitis)

Tendinitis is an inflammatory response of the tendon(s) to impingement. The condition is reversible at this stage.

- Initially the patient complains of a dull ache following an activity, but this progresses to pain during the performance of an activity.
- Somatic referred pain is experienced in the C5 segment.
- Sleep is affected.
- There is a painful arc of abduction (Figure 3–5) between 60° and 120° (Hawkins & Abrams, 1987).
- A positive impingement sign is present: pain is manifested when the greater tuberosity is forced against the anterior inferior surface of the acromion during forward flexion.
- There may be some restriction of motion because of pain but the patient can be encouraged to move through it and there is no loss of passive range.
- There is tenderness on palpation over the affected tendon(s).

### Stage Two (Thickening and Fibrosis)

The second stage can be recognized by the fact that conservative treatment and decreased activity do not reverse the process.

- Aching becomes a major problem, disturbing sleep and interfering with daily activities.
- Active and passive movements are limited.
- Soft tissue crepitus, brought about by scarring in the subacromial space, is present.
- There is a catching sensation at about 100° when the arm moves downwards from elevation. This is thought to be caused by entrapment of scar tissue beneath the acromion (Hawkins & Abrams, 1987).

### Stage Three (Rotator Cuff Tears, Biceps Rupture, and Bony Changes)

Stage three is the chronic stage of the disease. Some of the clinical features described above persist and the following features are also present:

- there is an increased restriction in the range of motion, and weakness of the affected muscles is evident;
- atrophy is present in the region of the affected muscles;
- bony changes are evident on the head of the humerus. Osteophytes are present on the inferior surface of the acromion and may involve the coracoacromial ligament.

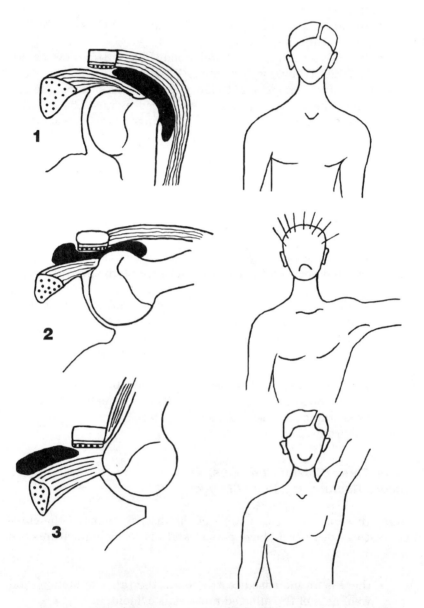

**Figure 3–5.** The painful arc: (1) arm at the side with no pain, (2) pain experienced at 90° of abduction, and (3) no pain beyond 120° of elevation through abduction.

## Treatment Guidelines

### Stage One

The aim of stage one treatment is to detect the condition in its earliest stage (tendinitis) and to prevent progression to the later stages. The following are useful approaches:

- rest from irritating activities;
- small range oscillatory movements grades 1 and 2 (Maitland, 1991) to the head of the humerus to relieve pain;
- ice and ultrasound to decrease pain and swelling;
- frictions across the tendon(s) for mobilization and prevention of adhesion formation;
- stretching and strengthening exercises as pain permits.

### Stages Two and Three

The aim of treatment in stage two and stage three is to maintain pain-free functional activities by ensuring there is sufficient range of motion and strength to achieve these activities. Some of the approaches suggested above may be carried over to this stage but the emphasis is on maintenance of a functional range of motion and strength.

The above stages overlap, as the disease can be a continuous process.

## Surgical Intervention

Surgery consists of a decompression procedure and it focuses on removing the structures against which the soft tissue structures are impinging; usually this involves removal of the anterior one third of the acromion (acromioplasty) and associated osteophytes.

*Note:* Patte (1990) has pointed out that impingement can occur between the coracoid process and the lesser tuberosity, in which case an acromioplasty will be ineffective.

## ROTATOR CUFF TEARS AND REPAIR

Ruptures of the rotator cuff muscles can develop over a period of time as a result of the repeated impingement process described previously, or suddenly as a result of a fall on the outstretched hand or in young people as a result of athletic activity. However, in older people they are much more common in the chronic form, resulting from attrition caused by degeneration (R.J. Neviaser, 1987b).

## A. ACUTE TEARS

An acute tear can be partial or complete and in young people it is often difficult to determine the exact state of the cuff since pain is quite often severe and the patient is unable to raise the arm sideways because of it. Differentiation clinically is dependent on whether the patient's attempt to raise the arm sideways results in a shoulder shrug (complete tear) or a positive drop arm test (partial tear) in which the patient is able to raise the arm sideways but is unable to maintain the position when minimal resistance is applied.

### Clinical Features

Partial and complete tears demonstrate the following characteristics:

- positive impingement sign;
- weakness when attempts are made to abduct or laterally rotate the arm;
- positive palm down abduction test (weakness against resistance at 60°);
- tenderness in the region of the greater tuberosity and bicipital groove.

### Surgical Procedure

A decompression procedure is performed by resecting the coracoacromial ligament and removing the anteroinferior part of the acromion (acromioplasty). The frayed edges of the torn cuff are removed and, utilizing sutures and drill holes in the bone and cuff, are replaced as close to their original position as possible.

## B. CHRONIC TEARS

Chronic tears are found in 90 per cent of patients, and usually occur in people in the fifth decade or later.

## Clinical Features

- The onset of pain is insidious, and made worse by using the arm in the overhead position.
- Sleep is often disturbed.
- The drop arm test may not be positive and when so is indicative of a massive tear.
- There is tenderness over the acromioclavicular joint.
- Movement is only slightly restricted.
- There is weakness of external rotation when compared to the sound side.
- Positive palm down abduction and impingement signs are present.
- Crepitus is evident.

### Differential Tests

Since it is well known that conditions of the cervical spine can produce shoulder pain the cervical spine must be cleared as a possible cause. The section on the Upper Limb Tension Test later in this chapter describes a useful differential test.

## Treatment Guidelines

The main aim is relief of pain. The following procedures may be found useful:

- injections of steroids into the subacromial space (no more than three over a given time period);
- ice, ultrasound;
- gentle range of motion exercises and gentle stretching.

*Note:* Vigorous strengthening exercises, particularly above shoulder level, are likely to aggravate the condition.

Operative treatment as described previously is undertaken only if conservative approaches fail, but restoration of range of motion is not as predictable as in the younger age group.

*Note:* It is important that a diagnosis be made as early as possible and an injection of lidocaine into the subacromial space to relieve the pain may be necessary. If surgical repair for a complete tear is to be carried out it should be done within 3 weeks of injury for the best results to be achieved (R.J. Neviaser, 1987b). However, the results of repair of rotator cuff tears have been difficult to compare because of the lack of a classification system. Patte (1990) has developed such a system.

## CALCIFIED SUPRASPINATUS TENDON

Calcium is known to develop in relation to certain joint structures in the body, but is common in the subacromial structures. The supraspinatus tendon is the most susceptible to calcification, probably attributable to the fact that it is prone to degeneration in the region of the avascular critical zone of the tendon (Kessel, 1982). The calcific mass consists of a calcium substance which resembles either a milky emulsion or a granular form (Gartner & Simons, 1990). The former occurs during the very painful acute stage and the latter during the chronic stage.

### Clinical Features

- The presence of calcium may not give rise to painful symptoms but frequently does.
- The pain that accompanies the acute stage of calcification is extremely intense because of the acute inflammatory reaction that is present. This acute inflammatory reaction has been described as a "chemical abscess" (Kessel, 1982). The patient may say that the pain brings tears to the eyes.
- The painful arc is present, if the pain permits movement of the arm.
- In the subacute state the calcium can become resorbed or it penetrates the subacromial bursa and a bursitis results. In either case there is a relief of pain because of the reduction of pressure over a limited area. If, however, the bursa becomes involved a bursitis results which produces swelling in the subacromial region.

### Treatment Guidelines

Ultrasound may assist the process of resorption but needling and curetting of the deposit are often necessary (Ellman, 1990).

## ADHESIVE CAPSULITIS

Adhesive capsulitis is a condition in which there is a spontaneous onset of shoulder pain followed by increasingly severe restriction of all glenohumeral movements. It has been loosely termed "frozen shoulder" but T.J. Neviaser (1987b) has pointed out that this is a misnomer since it is possible to have a stiff and painful shoulder without involvement of the inferior fold of the capsule which is a key feature of adhesive capsulitis.

## Etiology

Although the condition has been in existence for more than 100 years the cause is unknown. However, there are certain facts of etiological significance that are known and these are listed below.

1. Adhesive capsulitis occurs in both men and women between the ages of 40–60 years and is a little more common in women than in men.
2. The non-dominant shoulder is affected more often than the dominant shoulder.
3. There appears to be evidence that the condition is more common in patients with cervical spondylosis, cardiac ischemia, and diabetes.

## Pathology

There are three phases to the disease: pain, stiffness, and recovery (Baslund, Thomsen, & Jensen, 1990).

There is a suggestion of an inflammatory process.

There is a reduction in the capacity of the joint capsule largely caused by intra-articular adhesions particularly in the inferior joint recess.

The joint capsule is fibrosed and friable and there is evidence of altered biochemical composition.

## Clinical Features

The stages in adhesive capsulitis are overlapping.

- The condition often begins to develop with pain in the deltoid region at night; this symptom is rather similar to that experienced in the impingement syndrome. The pain increases in intensity over the next few days, sleep is disturbed, and there is also pain at rest. The pain is probably caused by synovitis. This phase can last between 10 and 36 weeks (Baslund et al. 1990).
- The onset of restriction of range of motion is associated with the pain, and the loss of range increases as the pain persists. The restriction is evident by about 2–3 weeks after onset.
- Pain gradually recedes over the next few weeks as the synovitis subsides, but the joint becomes increasingly stiff. Although there is no pain at rest, attempts to move the arm will produce pain. This period lasts between 4 and 12 months (Baslund et al. 1990).

*Note:* The capsular pattern is present in that lateral rotation is more limited than abduction which is more limited than medial rotation.

## Treatment Guidelines

Since patients are usually seen by the therapist when joint restriction is established, the following approach to treatment is frequently adopted:

- Passive mobilization of the scapulothoracic mechanism and glenonumeral joint is followed by exercises; the patient is taught auto assisted, free active, isometric, and resisted exercises to perform at home.
- It is explained to the patient that recovery can take several months.
- Manipulation of the shoulder under anesthetic is carried out if conservative measures fail.

## THE UPPER LIMB TENSION TEST (ULTT)

It was stated earlier in this chapter that problems with the cervical spine can refer pain to the shoulder; indeed, shoulder pain may be the only symptom of which the patient complains. If, under these circumstances, the shoulder is treated the patient's symptoms will not improve.

It is known that structures at the site of referred pain can develop secondary pathological changes such as restriction of movement and pain that can mask the fact that the cervical spine is the culprit (Wells, 1982). The longer the shoulder pathology has been in existence the more difficult it is to bring about a reversal of symptoms by treating the cervical spine alone, and it becomes necessary to treat both areas.

The ULTT was developed by Elvey (1979, 1986) and modified by Kenneally, Rubenach, and Elvey (1988) in an attempt to differentiate between the cervical spine and the glenohumeral joint as the cause of the patient's shoulder problem. The test exerts a longitudinal traction force on the trunks of the peripheral nerves and the nerve roots of the cervical spine. If the shoulder symptoms are reproduced the problem is arising from the cervical spine or from a component of the latter (Kenneally et al., 1988).

Pathological changes in the cervical spine invariably lead to adhesions and fibrous tissue formation around the nerve roots. If this happens the mobility of the roots is restricted and they become more susceptible to tensile stresses. During the performance of the ULTT a progressive stretch is applied to the peripheral nerve trunks with each stage of the test. This stretch is emphasized at the level of the nerve roots in the cervical spine; if the patient's shoulder pain is reproduced during the performance of the test it follows that pathology in the cervical spine is wholly or partly responsible for the patient's shoulder pain.

In order to avoid stretching structures other than the nerve root, for example muscles, the component movements of the test are taken to the end of the pain-free range only; for instance, if shoulder pain appears or increases when the elbow is extended fully then the elbow is moved into a pain-free range of extension since the pain is probably caused by stress on a soft tissue structure other than the nerve root. At the stage of adding the final component of wrist and finger extension the limb should be pain free. The addition of the last component puts maximum stretch on the upper nerve roots and if the cervical spine is responsible for the patient's shoulder pain that pain will be reproduced.

## Stages and Technique of the ULTT

### Position of the Patient

The patient lies in the supine position with the side to be tested close to the edge of the plinth. The test is described for the right side.

The test is performed in three component parts and as each part is performed the patient's pain is assessed.

The three component parts are:

1. shoulder abduction, extension and lateral rotation;
2. full supination of the forearm followed by extension of the elbow;
3. wrist and finger extension.

### Position of the Therapist

The therapist half sits on the plinth at the side of the patient close to the right shoulder and facing the patient.

The therapist's right hand embraces the top of the shoulder girdle with the fingers curling beneath the posterior aspect.

- *Movement One:* The therapist abducts the arm to approximately 110° or where maximum tension is exerted since this is going to vary from patient to patient. The therapist is careful to maintain the mid-range position to avoid any unnecessary stretch on the structures of the shoulder. The arm is then extended to about 10° beyond the coronal plane (the anterior capsule of the shoulder should not be stressed), and laterally rotated to approximately 60°. The position should be comfortable for the patient and hence movements should not be pushed to the limit. The patient is questioned about any shoulder pain.
- *Movement Two:* The therapist fully supinates the arm and slowly extends the elbow. The patient's arm is supported by the therapist's thigh just proximal to the elbow. Once again the patient is questioned regarding shoulder pain.
- *Movement Three:* If the patient is still not complaining of shoulder pain then the wrist and fingers are extended. The right hand of the therapist moves down to support the elbow and keep it in full extension as the left hand gently extends the wrist and fingers.

When Movement Three has been performed there is maximum stretch on the peripheral nerve or nerve roots. Again the patient is asked about shoulder pain. If the pain has not been reproduced then the test can be repeated with the addition of one of the sensitizing movements discussed below, for example, side flexion of the cervical spine to the left.

As mentioned previously there are certain stretch responses which are quite normal and must be expected. The patient will experience a stretch across the anterior aspect of the shoulder, a deep stretch sensation across the anterior aspect of the elbow, and tingling in the C6 and C7 dermatomes in the hand. **Only if the patient's shoulder pain is reproduced is the ULTT positive.**

The test is not infallible and a positive result is dependent upon there being the type of pathology present in the cervical spine that compromises the nerve roots. Consequently, it is possible to have a problem in the cervical spine that is causing the shoulder pain, but that will not result in a positive ULTT.

Finally the technique described is the basic technique. Sensitivity to the test can be increased by placing the contralateral arm in abduction and lateral rotation or the cervical spine in almost any pain-free position before the ULTT is applied. Side flexion of the cervical spine to the contralateral side is commonly used.

## ANTERIOR SHOULDER INSTABILITIES

Anterior shoulder instabilities are present if there is weakness in one or more of the anterior supporting structures, for instance subscapularis, and the humerus slips forwards and backwards in the glenoid cavity giving rise to pain.

A person with an unstable shoulder is vulnerable to injury, particularly subluxation (partial malalignment of the articular surfaces) or dislocation (complete separation of the articular surfaces). Athletes who depend on rhythmic and rapid coordination of the shoulder can be severely disabled (Rowe, 1990). O'Brien, Warren, and Schwartz (1987) have stated that although shoulder instability is a fairly common problem it has escaped notice in its milder forms. They make a distinction between laxity (loose ligaments), which occurs normally in varying degrees, and instability which they describe as a clinical entity.

## A. ANTERIOR DISLOCATION

Anterior dislocation occurs when the head of the humerus disengages completely from the glenoid cavity by moving anteriorly. Anterior dislocation of the shoulder is the complete separation of the articular surfaces of the glenohumeral joint caused by indirect or, less commonly, direct forces.

## Mechanism of Injury

Indirect forces caused by a fall on the hand and involving abduction, external rotation, and extension are the most common mechanisms of injury. Dislocation attributable to direct forces is much less common. As a result of the dislocation the head of the humerus is displaced beneath the coracoid.

## Clinical Features

- The arm is held in the abducted position.
- Pain and spasm may be considerable, and can prevent movement.
- The shoulder will not present with its normal rounded contour, but will appear squared off when viewed from the front.
- The acromion is more prominent than normal.

## Method of Reduction

Reduction can be achieved utilizing the Kocher method. This involves traction when the arm is slowly rotated externally to 90°. The arm will usually relocate at 90° of external rotation with a "clunking noise." If this does not occur the arm is adducted so that the flexed elbow is across the chest, and internally rotated so that the patient's hand is across the chest. The last two movements can be performed quite quickly. Another method involves placing the patient in the prone position with a sandbag beneath the clavicle and the shoulder free of the plinth; the arm is allowed to hang down over the side of the plinth. The shoulder can reduce spontaneously within the hour.

## Treatment Guidelines

A sling is worn for approximately 4–6 weeks after reduction. Rehabilitation focuses on strengthening the internal rotators, particularly subscapularis. Pectoralis major and coracobrachialis also receive attention. Abduction to 90° with lateral rotation is not allowed during the early part of the exercise program because subscapularis is not working with the same mechanical effect with the arm in this position.

## B. RECURRENT ANTERIOR DISLOCATION

## Mechanisms of Injury

The causes of recurrent anterior dislocation are:

* traumatic redislocation;
* daily dislocations during sleep, showering, and other activities.

The traumatic redislocations occur with repeatedly less trauma. The non-traumatic redislocations can either be voluntary or involuntary. Patients will report that they can make their shoulder pop out and back with no discomfort. This is sometimes called habitual dislocation (McRae, 1981). However, this could lead to a state where the shoulder pops out without the patient's help and with discomfort.

## Treatment

Usually, following an anterior dislocation, any damage to the capsule repairs spontaneously and the dislocation does not recur (Apley, 1973). However, if there is tearing of the capsule and disruption of the glenoid labrum (Bankart lesion) recurrence is very likely and surgical intervention involving reattachment of these structures becomes necessary. Another common surgical approach is the Putti-Platt (or a modification of the Putti-Platt). This involves reefing the subscapularis over the anterior part of the joint to deliberately restrict lateral rotation. Immobilization follows for a period of approximately 4 weeks.

## POSTERIOR SHOULDER INSTABILITIES

Posterior instabilities are not nearly as common as anterior shoulder instabilities, being present in approximately 2–4 per cent of patients presenting with unstable shoulders (Schwartz, Warren, O'Brien, & Fronek, 1987).

## A. POSTERIOR DISLOCATION

## Mechanism of Injury

Indirect forces that combine flexion, adduction and internal rotation are commonly the cause of posterior dislocation.

## Clinical Features

* The patient complains of pain and presents with the arm held in adduction and internal rotation.

- The coracoid process appears prominent.
- There is a bulge posteriorly.
- Movements are restricted because of pain in the arm.

## Method of Reduction

The patient is relaxed in the supine position and the following movements are tried in sequence:

- Lateral traction, in a position of 90° of abduction, external rotation (to relax the posterior capsule), and pressure in a postero-anterior (P/A) direction to relocate the head of the humerus.

## B. RECURRENT POSTERIOR DISLOCATION

Recurrent posterior shoulder instabilities are treated similarly to the anterior shoulder dislocations using the Bankart or modified Putti-Platt procedures. However, in the latter, the infraspinatus is reefed rather than the subscapularis.

## MULTIDIRECTIONAL INSTABILITIES

Multidirectional instabilities caused by general joint laxity are also fairly common. Alleviation of the patient's pain is a prime consideration. Isometric exercises and isotonic exercises within a limited range are implemented to produce functional motion (Jobe, Moynes, & Brewster, 1987).

## MYOFASCIAL TRIGGER POINTS

Myofascial trigger points were first identified by Dr. Janet Travell, and the following information is adapted from Travell and Simons (1983).

Active trigger points (TP's) are circumscribed areas of hyperirritability in a taut band of muscle or fascia. They are tender when compressed and can give rise to referred pain, the pattern of which is consistent with the site of origin of the trigger point. TP's can also cause autonomic phenomena. Latent TP's give rise to pain only when examined by palpation but their presence may be responsible for weakness of a muscle or joint restriction. They can become activated, for example, by overuse.

# Etiology

Trigger points are activated directly by:

- direct trauma;
- active overload;
- fatigue caused by sustained contractions or excessive repetitive activities;
- chilling (cold, damp, or a draft).

Trigger points are activated indirectly by:

- arthritic joints;
- emotional distress;
- visceral disease.

The greater the exercise tolerance of a muscle the less is the tendency to develop TP's or to activate latent areas.

# Clinical Features

- Normal muscles do not contain TP's or taut bands of muscle fibers, so TP's are present in muscles that have lost their extensibility or have otherwise become impaired.
- Individuals of either sex can develop TP's.
- They are a common source of musculoskeletal pain in childhood.
- The possibility of developing active TP's increases with age into the most active middle years, for example, 31–50 years.

### Signs and Symptoms

- Pain referred from a TP (Figure 3–6) is frequently non-segmental in its distribution. It does not include the whole segment and may include parts of additional segments. It is described as a dull, deep ache.
- The discomfort experienced can be moderate or excruciating and is related to the hyperirritability of the TP rather than the size of the muscle.
- Pain is increased if the TP is compressed.

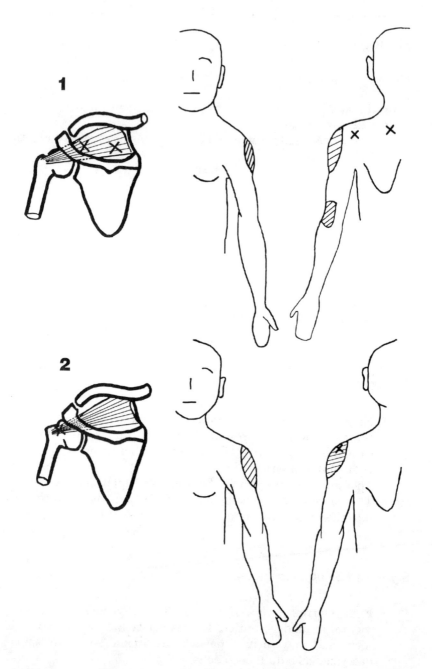

**Figure 3–6.** Trigger points for supraspinatus showing primary areas of pain referral (1) within the muscle and (2) within the tendon (adapted from Travell & Simons, 1983).

## How to Recognize a TP

1. There is a history of a sudden or gradual onset of pain following overload stress.
2. A palpable band of fibers within a muscle can be detected.
3. There is an increase in pain with compression of the TP.
4. There are characteristic patterns of pain produced that are associated with certain muscles.
5. If the TP is snapped between the fingers a local twitch response is produced.

*Note:* Numbers 4 and 5 above confirm the presence of a TP. Number 3 must be present for a diagnosis to be made, but by itself is inconclusive.

## Features Common to All Muscles

- Knowledge of the referred pain pattern identifies the muscle.
- Action of that muscle reveals which movements and stress situations are likely to activate and perpetuate the trigger points.
- A knowledge of the functional relationship of muscles helps to identify other muscles likely to develop TP's because of the interactive mechanical stress.

## Perpetuating Factors

Factors that perpetuate the problem may include:

1. mechanical stresses, for example poor posture, skeletal asymmetry, overuse activities;
2. nutritional inadequacies such as vitamins $B_1$, $B_6$, $B_{12}$ and C;
3. metabolic and endocrine inadequacies, for example hypometabolism or any condition which impairs muscle metabolism;
4. chronic infections caused by viral or bacterial diseases.

# Treatment Guidelines

The "stretch and spray" sequence as outlined below is an effective means of treating a TP in a single muscle (Travell & Simons, 1983).

1. The patient is seated in a comfortable, relaxed position.
2. One end of the muscle must be anchored so that pressure can be applied to passively stretch it.
3. The first sweep of a vapocoolant spray (Fluori-Methane is preferred) is applied before any stretch pressure is applied.
4. A jet stream, not a diffuse mist, of vapocoolant spray is applied in parallel sweeps in one direction, first over the entire length of the muscle including the referred pain zone. After each sweep the muscle is stretched.
5. The stretch and spray sequence can be repeated until full muscle length is achieved, **but any given area of skin should be covered only two or three times before rewarming.** Immediate application of a warm hot pack rewarms the skin and helps the muscle to relax.
6. After the skin has been rewarmed stretch and spray can be repeated.
7. Several cycles of full active range of motion complete one stretch and spray treatment of that muscle.

In addition to these treatments it is imperative that the patient be taught a stretching program to do at home, and be educated in the appropriate use of muscles to avoid overuse.

## SUPRASCAPULAR NERVE DISORDER

The suprascapular nerve is susceptible to injury, irritation, or entrapment in the suprascapular notch. It is involved more often than is generally thought and should be considered as a source of shoulder pain and weakness. It is derived from C5 and C6 nerve roots; it innervates the spinati muscles and provides sensory innervation to the acromioclavicular joint and the posterior capsule of the shoulder (Corrigan & Maitland, 1983).

### Mechanism of Injury

The most common cause of suprascapular nerve disorder appears to be compression of the nerve as it passes through the suprascapular notch beneath the transverse or suprascapular ligament.

Overuse of the scapulothoracic mechanism can create traction on the nerve; this is particularly so in hyperprotraction of the scapula (Rask, 1977), or in hyperprotraction combined with horizontal adduction of the glenohumeral joint (Skurja & Monlux, 1985). Wells (1985) has found that suprascapular nerve entrapment is not uncommon in pitchers suffering from prolonged shoulder pain.

Trauma sustained, for example, in a motor vehicle accident can damage the nerve.

## Clinical Features

Pain, often severe, is experienced in the posterolateral aspect of the shoulder and may radiate into the arm. It may be difficult to localize, but it can be increased by local pressure over the suprascapular notch or by passive hyperprotraction of the scapula combined with horizontal adduction of the glenohumeral joint.

There may be weakness and even atrophy of the spinati muscles, particularly if the condition is prolonged.

## Treatment

The following approaches may prove beneficial:

- rest;
- education and correction of the irritating activity;
- strengthening exercises for the spinati.
- An injection of a local anesthetic and corticosteroid may be necessary.

If none of the above are effective, resection of the transverse ligament of the scapula as a decompression procedure may be necessary.

*Note:* This condition may be overlooked or confused with a problem involving the rotator cuff muscles.

## SUMMARY

The component joints of the shoulder complex were listed and it was noted that they are interdependent and interrelated. Problems associated with this complex are common; however, it was pointed out that pain in the shoulder region often stems from the cervical spine and that a careful assessment is necessary to rule out the cervical spine as the cause of shoulder pain. The conditions discussed were done so in a proximal to distal order commencing with Acromioclavicular Injuries and, specifically, the different degrees of acromio-clavicular sprain. Common problems involving the muscles of the rotator cuff were described under the different stages of the Impingement Syndrome. An explanation was given regarding the vulnerability to injury of the tendon of supraspinatus and the biceps tendon. Adhesive Capsulitis, another common problem involving the glenohumeral joint, was discussed. Although the ULTT is not a specific disorder it was included in this chapter since it is recognized as a means of differentiating between shoulder pain arising from the cervical spine and that stemming from the glenohumeral joint. The chapter ended with a discussion on Shoulder Instabilities, Myofascial Trigger Points, and Suprascapular Nerve Entrapment.

# CHAPTER 4

# The Elbow, Wrist, and Hand

Functionally the elbow, wrist, and hand are closely related. The elbow, like the arm and forearm, plays an important role in placing the wrist and hand in space so that the functions of the hand can be performed. Many of the muscles controlling the wrist and hand movements arise from the elbow region, thus reinforcing the functional relationship. It is for this reason that these three mobile structures and their disorders will be discussed in this chapter.

## THE ELBOW

The elbow is the most proximal of the complex of the related joints; the pertinent anatomy and the disorders affecting this joint will be discussed first.

## FUNCTIONAL ANATOMY

The articulating surfaces that form the elbow joint are discussed first followed by a brief description of the muscles controlling the joint; finally there is a review of the collateral ligaments.

### Joints

The elbow is a compound synovial hinge joint consisting of the **humeroulnar** and the **humeroradial** joints. In the former the trochlea of the humerus, which is deeper in its medial part, articulates with the trochlear notch of the ulna. However, complete congruence is not present between the two articulating surfaces; the hinge movement is accompanied by the "screw home" mechanism and conjunct rotation (Warwick & Williams, 1973). Consequently there are 5° of ulnar external rotation during full extension and 5° of internal rotation during initial elbow flexion (Tullos & Bryan, 1985).

In the humeroradial joint the concave surface of the head of the radius articulates with the capitulum of the humerus. Closely associated with these joints, in the elbow complex, is the superior radioulnar joint and, distally, the inferior radioulnar joint. Flexion and extension take place in the humeroulnar and humeroradial joints and the humeroradial joint also facilitates pronation and supination, which occur in the radioulnar joints.

If the arm is placed at the side of the body with the elbow extended and the forearm supinated it will be seen that the elbow is in a valgus position of between 10–15°; this angle is even greater in women. This valgus position is called the **"carrying angle"** and it disappears when the elbow is in full flexion when a varus position is assumed. Tullos and Bryan (1985) have demonstrated that this change of position from valgus in extension to varus in flexion is caused by a trochlear slope of 15° from the lateral to medial side.

## Muscles

The muscles of the arm and the forearm are enclosed by fascial sheaths. The fascial sheaths of the arm are derived from the brachial fascia and those of the forearm are derived from the antebrachial fascia, which is continuous above with the brachial fascia. Blood vessels and nerves enter and exit the sheaths through apertures. It will be seen later that these fascial enclosures can cause problems under certain circumstances.

The muscles producing **flexion** of the elbow are **brachialis, biceps brachii**, and **brachioradialis**. The contribution these muscles make to the movement of elbow flexion varies. Brachialis is the main flexor and it functions effectively in both the supinated and pronated positions of the forearm. Biceps brachii is the main supinator of the forearm but it functions as a flexor in any position if the load is large enough. Brachioradialis functions effectively when the forearm is in the mid-position or fully pronated.

The triceps muscle is **the** extensor of the elbow. As its name suggests it arises from three heads, the long head, the lateral head, and the medial head. The latter is active whenever elbow extension takes place; the long head and the lateral head only become active when elbow extension occurs against resistance.

Arising from the anterior surfaces of the medial and lateral epicondyles of the humerus respectively are the common flexor tendon and the common extensor tendon. The muscles arising from these tendons control the movements of the wrist and hand. Their contribution to the elbow is to assist the **medial** and **lateral collateral ligaments** in maintaining medial and lateral stability.

## Medial Collateral Ligament

The medial collateral ligament is a thick triangular-shaped band consisting of anterior and posterior parts that are connected by a much thinner intermediate portion. The anterior and posterior surfaces of the ligament attach proximally to the anterior and posterior surfaces of the medial epicondyle. Distally, the anterior portion is attached to the medial margin of the coronoid process and the posterior part to the medial margin of the olecranon (Warwick & Williams, 1973). Tullos and Bryan (1985) have pointed out that the anterior part of the ligament is taut throughout the entire range of flexion and functions throughout the entire range of elbow motion; consequently it is the major restraint against a valgus stress. In contrast, the posterior part of the ligament is taut in flexion and lax in extension and does not contribute much to medial stability. It has been shown that severance of this part of the medial collateral ligament does not produce instability providing the anterior portion is intact (Tullos & Bryan, 1985). The ulnar nerve is closely associated with the posterior part of the medial collateral ligament (Figure 4–1).

## Lateral Collateral Ligament

The lateral collateral ligament attaches proximally to the lower part of the lateral epicondyle and distally to the annular ligament, which embraces the radial head. Some fibers are attached to the supinator crest on the ulna (Figure 4–2). The ligament is intimately associated with the supinator and extensor carpi radialis brevis muscles. A condition involving the latter will be discussed next.

## LATERAL EPICONDYLITIS ("TENNIS ELBOW")

Many different causes for lateral epicondylitis have been described but the most popular one is that it is due to an overuse injury affect-

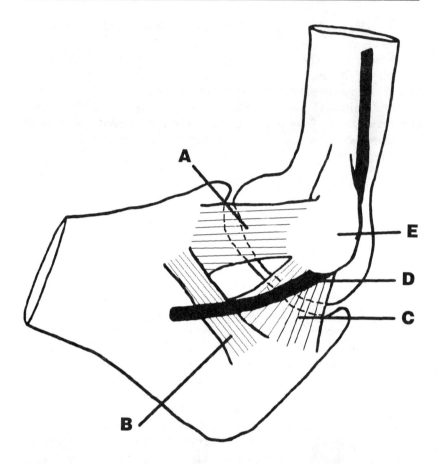

**Figure 4–1.** The medial collateral ligament of the elbow and its relationship to the ulnar nerve: (A) the anterior portion, (B) the oblique portion, (C) the posterior portion, (D) the ulnar nerve, and (E) the medial epicondyle.

ing the common extensor tendon, particularly the tendon of extensor carpi radialis brevis. The result is a painful inflammatory reaction at the origin of this muscle on the lateral epicondyle. Cyriax (1982) has identified the tenoperiosteal junction of the common extensor tendon as being the most common site of injury, and scar tissue as being the source of the patient's pain.

## Mechanism of Injury

Although in common terminology it is referred to as "tennis elbow" this condition can develop from most racket sports, or it may devel-

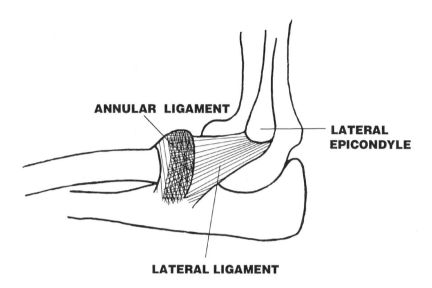

ANNULAR LIGAMENT

LATERAL
EPICONDYLE

LATERAL LIGAMENT

**Figure 4–2.** The lateral collateral ligament and the annular ligament.

op from repetitive movements completely unrelated to sporting activities. On occasion a single incident such as a poor backhand return in tennis may be responsible for the initiation of the inflammatory response; more commonly, it is brought about by overuse of a poorly conditioned wrist extensor mechanism (Wright, 1990). Repetitive use of radial wrist extension (such as in returning a backhand in tennis or gutting fowls in a chicken factory) is the prime cause of this problem.

## Clinical Features

The onset can be slow or sudden; the following signs and symptoms are present.

- The patient experiences pain over the anterior aspect of the lateral epicondyle on radial wrist extension; actions as simple as lifting a coffee cup or a telephone receiver may cause such pain that the patient drops the object.
- There is tenderness on palpation.
- The pain may extend down the extensor muscles to the back of the hand or up the arm.

- Resisted wrist extension with the elbow extended will increase the pain.
- The pain is frequently worse at night.

## Treatment Guidelines

The condition can be extremely challenging to treat. If it is caught in its early stages rest, ice and ultrasound, and frictions can be effective. Injections of hydrocortisone often bring some relief. The Mill's manipulation, as described by Cyriax (1982), has been successful in breaking down the painful scar tissue with relief of painful symptoms if the lesion is of the tenoperiosteal type located at the lateral epicondyle. The use of an arm band just distal to the lateral epicondyle has been shown to increase wrist extension and grip strength (Wadsworth, Nielson, Burns, Krull, & Thompson, 1989). Lee (1986) feels that the problem is many-faceted and requires a thorough evaluation of the upper quadrant in order to restore maximum function to the forearm. Kushner and Reid (1986) discuss two types of manipulations, one involving a varus thrust of the elbow and one restoring full extension (Mill's manipulation). They feel that the former is useful for "gapping" the joint and restoring joint play whereas the latter has its greatest effect on contractile elements. Nirschl (1973) provides a comprehensive program based on relieving the inflammatory effects; increasing forearm flexibility, power, and endurance; correcting faults in the backhand tennis stroke; and educating the player in the selection of tennis equipment in terms of the grip, weight of the racket, and related factors.

Curwin and Stanish (1984) have developed a very successful approach to the treatment of tennis elbow which, although it has some similarities with the regime advocated by Nirschl (1973), its focus is on the use of exercise. Some of the features of their approach which differ from those of Nirschl are presented below.

- Stretching of the wrist extensors with the forearm pronated, the elbow extended, and passively flexing the wrist with the opposite hand. The stretch is maintained for 30 seconds and is repeated 3 times.
- The patient's pronated forearm is supported on the treatment table with the elbow in extension, and the wrist and hand free in space. The patient is given a weight to hold—1 pound for a woman and 2 for a man in acute cases and up to

5 pounds in less severe cases. The weight is lowered and raised for 3 sets of 10 repetitions.
• Stretching is repeated and ice applied.

## GOLFER'S ELBOW

Golfer's elbow is a medial epicondylitis affecting the common flexor tendon arising from the medial epicondyle of the elbow. It is much less common than lateral epicondylitis and not as disabling.

## Mechanism of Injury

Golfer's elbow is caused by overuse of the wrist flexors as in the action of throwing in athletic activities. It also develops in the right elbow of the right handed golfer (Cyriax, 1982).

## Clinical Features

The symptomatology relates to the medial epicondyle but sudden, sharp, disabling pain is rare. The following symptoms may be present.

• Pain may be experienced at the medial epicondyle on resisted wrist flexion and possibly on resisted pronation.
• The pain rarely radiates.
• There is tenderness on palpation over the medial epicondyle.

## Treatment Guidelines

A similar regime to that presented for tennis elbow can be implemented here for the common flexors. The Mill's maneuver is not used.

## COLLATERAL LIGAMENT DISORDERS

The collateral ligaments and related structures of the elbow can be injured, as in the knee. However, as the elbow is a non-weight bearing joint, sprains are not as common or as severe as those of the knee. The medial collateral ligament, in particular the anterior portion, is the main defense against a valgus stress. Repetitive stresses to this ligament are common in overarm throwers; the results of these stresses will be discussed next.

## A. MEDIAL COLLATERAL LIGAMENT SPRAIN

In a careful analysis of the movements involved in pitching, Tullos and King (1973) determined that the elbow was subjected to severe valgus stress during the early part of the acceleration stage when the shoulder and elbow move forward leaving the forearm and hand behind. The repeated stresses result in damage to the soft tissue medial structures, the muscles, ligament, the ulnar nerve, and eventually to the joint itself. The damage to the medial collateral ligament will be discussed first.

## Mechanism of Injury

Any sport involving overarm throwing with rapid extension of the elbow can subject the medial aspect of the elbow to repeated stress (Jobe & Bradley, 1990).

## Clinical Features

Clinical features are elicited on the medial aspect of the elbow joint.

- There is a positive result to valgus stress testing with the elbow in 20–30° of flexion in that pain is experienced. Gapping will be present if the ligament is partially ruptured, producing instability.
- Swelling and tenderness are present on palpation over the medial ligament.
- The patient may experience the joint opening up during a throwing activity.
- There may be some limitation of extension.

## Treatment Guidelines

If the condition is discovered early it will respond to the rest, ice, analgesics, and anti-inflammatory (steroid) approach. However, faults in training and throwing need to be corrected.

Blackburn (1985) has developed a comprehensive off-season program which includes flexibility and strengthening exercises for the muscles of the upper extremity. Fauls (1985) has recommended techniques to warm up and cool down the throwing arm.

Severe instability, or failure of the conservative approach, will warrant surgical intervention.

*Note:* As indicated earlier the common flexor tendon can also be damaged. It can be distinguished from medial collateral instability by asking the athlete to perform wrist flexion against resistance; a painful result implicates the common flexor muscles.

# B. ULNAR NEURITIS

Earlier in this chapter the close relationship of the ulnar collateral ligament and the ulnar nerve was mentioned and this relationship will be pursued further now. The ulnar nerve enters the forearm through the cubital tunnel and lies on the the posterior part of the medial collateral ligament, which forms the floor of the tunnel.

## Mechanism of Injury

Anything which will diminish the size of the cubital tunnel, such as hypertrophy of associated structures, is likely to compress the ulnar nerve. It is subjected to traction forces during overarm throwing. Repetitive movements of elbow extension, with resultant valgus stresses, can cause entrapment or dislocation of the nerve (Jobe & Bradley, 1990).

## Clinical Features

Clinical features relate directly to the ulnar nerve.

- Pain is experienced at the medial aspect of the elbow.
- The pain may spread down the medial forearm. Tingling and numbness in the little and ring fingers are usually present.
- The patient may experience painful popping sensations during flexion and extension of the elbow, indicating that the nerve is dislocating.
- Pain is felt on palpation of the ulnar nerve at the elbow.

## Treatment Guidelines

In mild cases of ulnar neuritis the conservative regimen of rest, ice, analgesics, and anti-inflammatories may be sufficient. Transposing the ulnar nerve anteriorly is the surgical approach for more difficult cases.

## C. LATERAL COLLATERAL LIGAMENT SPRAIN

Sprains of the lateral collateral ligament are much less frequent and less severe. When they do arise it is as a result of direct trauma or a varus stress. The clinical features are similar to those of the medial collateral ligament sprain except that they relate to the lateral side; treatment guidelines are as for a medial collateral sprain.

*Note:* In addition to the conditions described above there are a number of associated joint problems which can develop as a result of the throwing action. These include traction spurs and loose bodies. Andrews and Wilson (1985) have reported on osteophytic formation on the olecranon as a result of impingement of this bone on the olecranon fossa. Tullos and Bryan (1985) point out that the humeroradial joint can be damaged because of impingement of the articular surfaces of the joint as a result of medial collateral instability.

## COMPARTMENTAL SYNDROME (COMPARTMENT SYNDROME)

In the early part of this chapter it was mentioned that the muscles of the upper extremity are enclosed in fascial compartments and that under certain conditions these can give rise to problems. The compartmental syndrome is the main problem arising from these enclosures. Matsen (1975) has defined the syndrome as one in which the tissues within the enclosed space are subjected to pressure to the extent that the circulation to those tissues is impaired and, as a result, their function is diminished. He points out that, because the muscles, vessels, and nerves are enclosed within this confined space, a significant functional disability can be the result. The condition can be present in both upper and lower extremities and in order to avoid repetition those syndromes in the lower extremity will be mentioned here. Turek (1984) has identified the most common sites of involvement as the volar compartment of the forearm, the anterior tibial compartment, the deep posterior compartment of the leg, and the peroneal compartment.

The classic example of compartmental syndrome in the upper extremity is **Volkmann's Ischemic Contracture**. This is a flexion deformity of the wrist and fingers caused by a contracture of the flexor muscles of the forearm as a result of ischemia (Figure 4–3). The cause of the ischemia is damage to, or blockage of, the brachial artery at the level of the elbow (see supracondylar fracture). It can also be caused by edema of the soft tissues of the forearm within a tight fascial compartment (Adams & Hamblen, 1990).

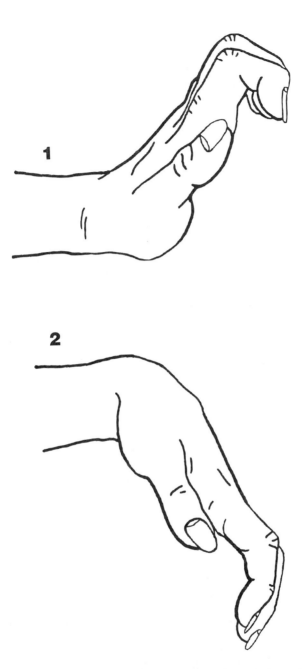

**Figure 4–3.** Volkmann's ischemic contracture: (1) flexor tightness with the wrist in extension, and (2) flexor laxity with the wrist in flexion (adapted from Kapandji, 1982).

In the lower extremity compartmental syndrome is commonly associated with a fracture or may be exercise-related in runners. Amendola and Rorabeck (1990) refer to it as "Chronic Exertional Compartment Syndrome" affecting the anterior compartment alone, or the anterior and posterior compartments, or the posterior compartment alone. It has also been described as an advanced stage of delayed onset muscle soreness (DOMS) in runners (Tiidus, 1990).

## Mechanisms Involved in the Increase in Pressure

Basically an increase in pressure on sensitive structures within the fascial compartments can be caused by:

- pressure from outside the compartment, which diminishes its size and thus increases the pressure within, such as a tight cast or dressing, or pressure from a tumor;
- pressure from within the compartment, brought about by an increase in volume within the confined space, for instance a hemorrhage or muscle hypertrophy due to weight lifting.

## Clinical Features

It is important that the clinical features be recognized as soon as possible because functional deficits can develop as a result of the ischemia within a short time. Patients with fractures, burns, or other trauma to the forearm or leg are considered to be at risk (Moore & Friedman, 1989). The clinical features have been well described by Matsen (1975), Turek (1984), and Moore and Friedman (1989); they are:

- inappropriate pain that is deep and poorly localized;
- paresthesia and numbness of distal parts;
- pain on passive stretching of affected muscles;
- progressive swelling and tenseness;
- tenderness on palpation over the affected compartment.

## Treatment Guidelines

The most effective treatment is identification of the patients at risk and early recognition of the condition before the effects of ischemia can cause irreversible changes. Conservative approaches, such as modification of activity, may be effective; otherwise, surgical decompression approaches such as fasciotomy should be implemented.

# THE WRIST AND HAND

In this section the functional role of the hand will be considered so that the conditions discussed later can be related to their functional effects. In addition specific pertinent anatomical structures will be described as they relate to the conditions under discussion.

## FUNCTIONAL CONSIDERATIONS OF THE WRIST AND HAND

The functional role of the joints of the upper extremity, including the wrist, is to position the hand in space so that it is able to perform its many significant functions. These functions include gross grasping movements and fine precision movements; these will be discussed next. The reader is encouraged to further explore these functional aspects as few people realize how disabling conditions affecting the hand can be; loss of the use of part of the hand is accompanied by a high anxiety level and other psychological ramifications.

The hand is used for gripping, grasping, holding, and for tactile functions. The hand grips most effectively with the wrist in extension, as indicated by flexion of the fingers when the wrist is extended. Conversely, with the wrist in flexion, the fingers will naturally extend.

## Gripping, Grasping, and Holding

Generally speaking the radial side of the hand is responsible for precision movements, such as the pinch grips and the chuck grip, and the ulnar side of the hand is responsible for the power grip. This can be demonstrated by asking someone to grip a pencil firmly between the index finger and thumb and it will be seen that it can easily be retrieved. If the pencil is held between the ring and little fingers and the palm the chances of retrieval are much reduced. Similarly, turning a key in a lock (involving a skill) is much easier utilizing the thumb and index finger than with any other combination of fingers or finger and thumb. It should also be noted that the index finger is able to function independently, whereas the other fingers are not able to do so.

## The Arches of the Hand

The arches of the hand (Figure 4–4) facilitate the functions by allowing the hand to embrace objects of various shapes and sizes. There are three arches associated with the hand (Kapandji, 1982)

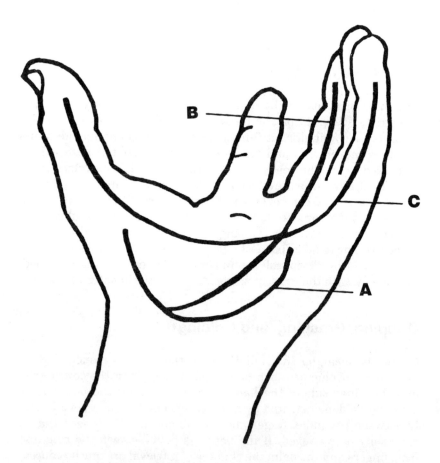

**Figure 4–4.** The arches of the hand: (A) the transverse arch, (B) the longitudinal arch, and (C) the oblique arch (adapted form Kapandji, 1982).

and all are located on the palmar surface. The **transverse arch** lies at the level of the wrist and is formed by the concavity of the carpal bones. Distally it extends to the arch formed by the metacarpal heads. Part of the **longitudinal arch** forms the gutter of the transverse arch and passes through the lunate, capitate, and the third metacarpal. Other parts of the longitudinal arch correspond to the remaining fingers. Kapandji has identified the arch of the middle finger and that of the index finger as being the most significant components of the **longitudinal arch**. The most important components of the **oblique arch** are those connecting the thumb and index finger and the thumb and the little finger.

## The Role of the Thumb in the Function of the Hand

The role of the thumb is vital to the function of the hand; indeed it has been estimated that it is responsible for approximately 50 percent of hand function. Observation of the hand clearly indicates that the thumb is set at a 90° angle to the rest of the fingers. It will also be noted that the first carpometacarpal joint has the greatest range of motion because of the fact that it is a saddle joint (MacConaill & Basmajian, 1969). This motion is brought about by the muscles of the thenar eminence: namely the opponens pollicis, the abductor pollicis brevis, and the flexor pollicis brevis, which play a significant role in grip and grasp. The flexor pollicis brevis is very effective in gripping a firm handle, but its role is taken over by opponens pollicis when increased thumb abduction is required to grasp a plastic coffee mug (MacConaill & Basmajian, 1969).

The long flexors and extensors of the forearm work in conjunction with the intrinsic muscles of the hand to control the movements of the metacarpophalangeal and interphalangeal joints.

## Flexor Retinaculum (Transverse Carpal Ligament)

The flexor retinaculum is a strong band of fibrous tissue extending anteriorly across the carpal bones. Medially it is attached to the **pisiform** and the **hook of hamate** and laterally to the **scaphoid and trapezium** (Figure 4–5). It forms the roof of the **carpal tunnel**, through which pass the flexor tendons in their sheaths and the median nerve.

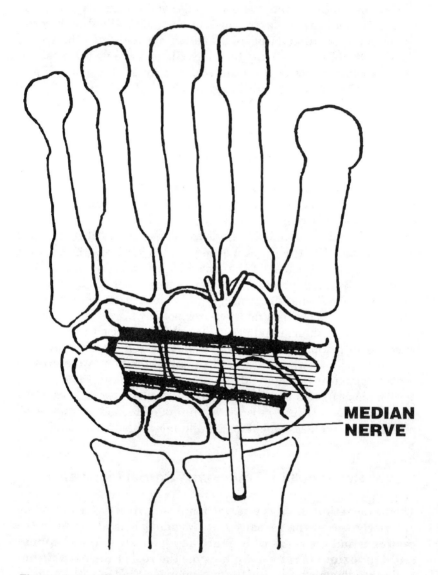

**Figure 4–5.** The median nerve passing beneath the flexor retinaculum (adapted from Cailliet, 1988).

## Flexor Tendon Sheaths

The flexor tendon sheaths extend from the distal palmar flexion crease to the distal phalanx (Figure 4–6). Surrounding these sheaths, at five levels, are annular pulley systems, which maintain the tendons in close contact with the bone. Without this system, particu-

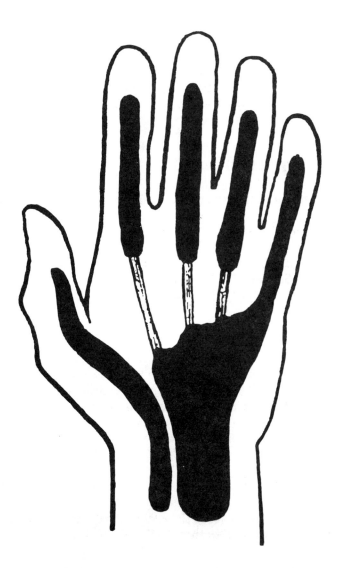

**Figure 4–6.** The flexor tendon sheaths (adapted from Netter, 1989).

larly in controlling the proximal phalanx and the middle phalanx, flexion of the fingers becomes inefficient. The blood supply of the flexor tendons is distributed segmentally along the tendons by vincula (Malick & Kasch, 1984).

## Palmar Aponeurosis

The palmar aponeurosis, located in the palm of the hand, is composed of fibrous tissue. It consists of a strong central part and weaker medial and lateral parts. The central part is triangular in shape and its apex is continuous with the flexor retinaculum; its base divides into four slips which pass distally to each finger. It is bound to the skin and covers the tendons of the flexor digitorum muscles. The medial and lateral parts cover the hypothenar eminence and thenar eminence respectively.

## DE QUERVAIN'S DISEASE

The extensor tendons of the wrist and fingers are enclosed in synovial sheaths representing six compartments. The first compartment, on the radial side of the hand, contains the tendons of abductor pollicis longus and extensor pollicis brevis. Although tenosynovitis can affect any of the synovial sheaths and their tendons, it commonly affects those in the first compartment at the level of the radial styloid; the condition is known as de Quervain's disease.

## Mechanism of Injury

The condition is probably an overuse syndrome of the abductor pollicis longus and extensor pollicis brevis, aggravated by their close proximity to the radial styloid. Activities such as wringing or continual use of a thumb pinch with wrist movements may be causative factors (Salter, 1983; Turek, 1984).

## Clinical Features

The clinical features relate to the radial side of the wrist at the level of the radial styloid and to the function of the hand.

- There is swelling and tenderness over the radial styloid.
- Movements of the thumb cause acute pain, particularly passive flexion of the thumb with ulnar deviation of the wrist (Finkelstein's test).
- Weakness of the thumb muscles occurs because of the pain.

## Treatment Guidelines

De Quervain's disease usually responds to rest, ultrasound, and/or a local injection of hydrocortisone. Surgically incising the tendon sheaths is advisable if there is severe disability. Rehabilitation focuses on restoring the normal function of the thumb and hand.

## CARPAL TUNNEL SYNDROME

The roof of the carpal tunnel is formed by the flexor retinaculum and the floor is formed by the carpal bones (Figure 4–5). The tendon of flexor pollicis longus, the tendons of flexor digitorum superficialis and profundus, and the median nerve are all contained within the tunnel.

The condition is regarded by some as a compartmental syndrome (Matsen, 1975) and by others as a compression neuropathy.

## Etiology

Any lesion at the wrist which results in pressure within the tunnel can give rise to this condition, for example arthritis, fractures, or tenosynovitis of the flexor tendons. The latter is probably the result of an overuse syndrome of the flexor tendons in industry or of a repetitive movement such as typing or knitting. The volume within a fairly confined space is increased resulting in pressure on the median nerve.

## Clinical Features

The symptomatology of the condition is related to the compression of the median nerve within the tunnel.

- There is numbness, tingling, or burning pain in the thumb, index and middle fingers, and the radial half of the ring finger; this distribution may vary, with the middle finger most frequently involved.
- The patient is usually awakened in the early hours of the morning by the discomfort; the hand feels swollen and heavy because of venous engorgement.
- In an attempt to relieve the discomfort the patient will shake the hand over the side of the bed, or get up and walk around.
- The movements of the hand may become clumsy.
- Weakness of the muscles of the thenar eminence will occur if the condition is long-standing, resulting in a flattened appearance of the thenar eminence.
- There is tenderness on palpation over the flexor retinaculum, and percussion over the median nerve produces a tingling sensation in the hand (positive Tinel's test).
- Initially the patient may say that the discomfort or numbness affects all the fingers in the hand, but when asked to take note of whether the little finger is involved the response is negative.

## Treatment Guidelines

The treatment is related to the cause. If the cause is an inflammatory reaction of the tendon sheaths then a modification of activities, rest, and an injection of hydrocortisone may be beneficial. If the cause is attributable to increased pressure from outside the compartment, as for example with a fracture, or if conservative measures are not successful, a decompression procedure involving division of the flexor retinaculum is in order.

## DUPUYTREN'S DISEASE

In Dupuytren's disease the palmar aponeurosis shortens and thickens resulting in a nodular formation in the palm of the hand (Figure 4–7) usually in line with the ring finger (Howard, 1959; McFarlane & Albion, 1984). The disease is progressive (though not on a predictable basis) and can result in tight cords extending from the nodule to the fingers; the result is flexion contractures (Dupuytren's contracture) of the ring and little fingers involving the metacarpophalangeal (MCP) joints (Figure 4–8), and sometimes also the

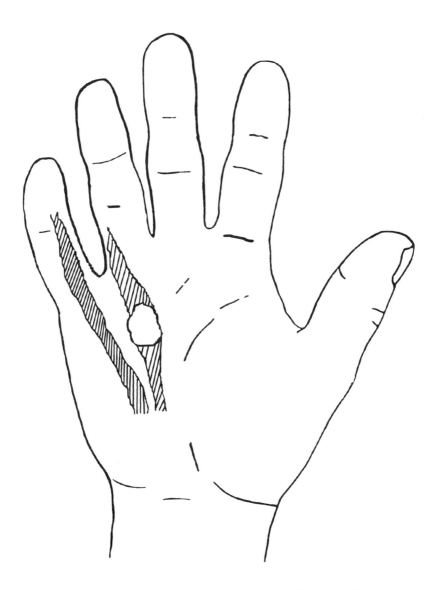

**Figure 4–7.** Tightness of the palmar fascia with nodular formation in Dupuytren's disease.

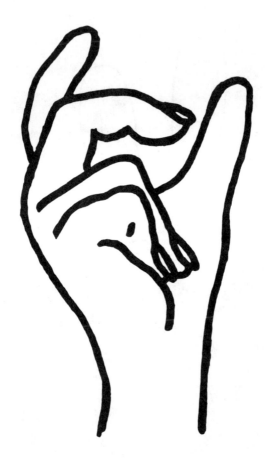

**Figure 4–8.** Clinical manifestation of Dupuytren's disease (adapted from Kapandji, 1982).

proximal interphalangeal phalangeal (PIP) joints. Less commonly the thumb and web of the thumb become involved.

## Etiology

The cause is unknown. The greatest incidence is found in Northern Europeans and males are affected much more than females. It is much more common after the age of 65 years and is associated with alcoholism and diabetes (Hill & Hurst, 1989).

## Clinical Features

The clinical features develop over a period of time and are described beginning with the earliest signs and continuing to the established deformity.

* A nodular structure develops in the palm of the hand in line with the ring finger.
* The nodule may be tender on palpation initially but discomfort disappears.
* Other nodules develop followed by cord-like structures extending from the nodules into the fingers; these are more apparent on extension of the fingers.
* Where the fascial aponeurosis is attached to the skin, dimpling may occur, either as an early or late manifestation (Howard, 1959), and the skin looks dry and undernourished.
* Flexion deformities of the involved fingers develop at the MCP joints and PIP joints with, possibly, hyperextension of the distal interphalangeal joint.
* There is restriction of motion particularly in extension.

## Treatment Guidelines

Conservative treatment is ineffective and surgical intervention is necessary if the function of the hand is severely affected. The surgical approach varies and involves removal of part or all of the aponeurosis.

After surgery the hand is elevated to control edema. This is followed by the application of a finger extension splint, with Velcro attachments, and the patient is encouraged to regain full extension within 2 days by gradually tightening the Velcro straps.

Passive extension and active movements to regain flexion and extension of the fingers, under the supervision of a therapist, are an important aspect in restoration of normal movement (McFarlane & Albion, 1984).

## REFLEX SYMPATHETIC DYSTROPHY

Reflex sympathetic dystrophy is a condition in which the hand is characterized by severe pain, swelling, stiffness, and discoloration in a progressive manner. It is usually preceded by trauma at a joint proximal to that in which the condition occurs.

## Mechanism of Onset

The condition is considered to be caused by abnormal sympathetic reflex activity (Turek, 1984) following an upper extremity trauma such as a crushing injury, elective surgery, or a fracture or sprain.

## Clinical Features

The clinical features exist in three stages and have been well described by Lankford (1984).

### Stage 1

- This stage usually lasts 3 months.
- Pain, usually of a burning nature, is the dominant feature which increases throughout this stage.
- Pain increases with attempted motion.
- Swelling develops early on.
- Painful paresthesia to light touch may be present.
- Restricted wrist and finger motion is evident.
- Discoloration occurs; the part is either pale or cyanotic to begin but later becomes red.
- There is increased sweating, and coolness.
- Osteoporosis of the carpal bones develops in 3–5 weeks.
- The skin is shiny.

### Stage 2

- This stage extends to 9 months.
- Pain continues to increase as does the stiffness of the joints. The pain is aggravated by attempted movement.
- Swelling changes to edema.
- Redness, decreased sweating, and increased heat develop.
- Osteoporosis increases.
- Shiny skin continues to be present.

### Stage 3

- This stage extends to 2 years and beyond.
- Continuous pain begins to subside but pain on motion continues to exists.

- Periarticular thickening of the joints occurs.
- The hand is dry, cool, and pale.
- Trophic changes of skin and nails are apparent.

## Treatment Guidelines

### Mild Cases With Minimal Skin and Joint Changes

Apply heat with the hand in an elevated position, and carry out short but frequent exercise sessions in the elevated position. Gentle passive movements should be given within limits of pain. Treat the entire extremity—shoulder, elbow, wrist, and hand using the exercise regimen.

### Moderate Cases

A stellate ganglion block (at the level of C6-C7 vertebrae) is used to interrupt the abnormal sympathetic reflex. This prevents efferent sympathetic activity into the extremity. A satisfactory block will bring about an almost pain-free state, a generalized drying and warming, and a return to normal color in the extremity.

Exercises follow to restore strength and range.

## FLEXOR TENDON INJURIES

Injuries to the flexor tendon require specific anatomical knowledge and surgical and clinical expertise in the operative approach to treatment and rehabilitation.

## Mechanisms of Injury

Such injuries could result from lacerations from knives, broken glass, fractures, and similar trauma.

## Clinical Features

The clinical features relate directly to the site of injury and functions of the tendon.

- There is pain, swelling, and loss of motion. The latter may not be specifically evident and requires a detailed assessment procedure.
- As with other hand injuries there is anxiety on behalf of the patient related to the loss of function of the hand.

## Considerations Prior to Surgery

Although some of the anatomy related to flexor tendons was discussed earlier in this chapter it is appropriate to look at this a little more carefully in terms of the factors that need to be considered prior to surgery. The following is an adaptation of the anatomical considerations as outlined by Horner (1983).

### Circulation

The blood supply to the flexor tendons is via the **mesotendon** on the dorsal aspect of the tendon. The mesotendon is composed of alveolar tissue in the forearm and palm, but in the fingers there is a localized connecting system (the vincular system). The significance of this system is that, having nourished the flexor digitorum superficialis (FDS) at the PIP joint, the vincula longa continue on to nourish the flexor digitorum profundus (FDP) (Figure 4–9). If, however, the blood supply to the FDS is interrupted through trauma, the blood supply to the FDP will be affected. Interference in the circulation can result in the formation of adhesions which will prevent tendon gliding.

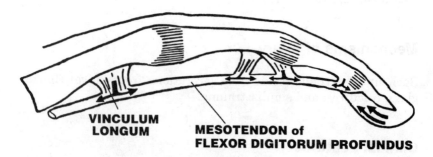

VINCULUM
LONGUM    MESOTENDON of
FLEXOR DIGITORUM PROFUNDUS

**Figure 4–9.** The blood supply to flexor digitorum profundus (adapted from Horner, 1983).

### Synovial Nutrition

There are no blood vessels on the palmar aspect. Nourishment is provided by the synovial fluid from the flexor tendon sheaths originating at the level of the distal palmar crease and terminating at the level of the distal phalanx. Cut flexor tendons can heal in synovial fluid from intact synovial membranes. If the tendon sheath is not damaged it helps to prevent adhesion formations.

### Pulley Function

An intact pulley system is very important to effective flexion of the interphalangeal joints, both from the mechanical and nutritional aspect. The gliding tendons must be held near the bone at the MCP joint or most of the tendon excursion will be taken up in flexion of the MCP joint with resultant loss of flexion at the PIP joints. Similarly an effective pulley must exist at the PIP joint in order to produce satisfactory flexion at the DIP joint.

### Tendon Repair

In order to ensure effective gliding a repair must be accurate. There must be no interference with the gliding of one FDS tendon on a FDP tendon, nor must there be interference in the gliding mechanism through the pulleys.

### Controlled Early Motion

Although it is virtually impossible to prevent some adhesion formation, with accurate repair of the tendon and sheath it can be minimized by early **controlled** motion.

## Treatment Guidelines

Several post-surgical programs have been developed based upon the principle of **controlled passive flexion** of the affected tendon. These are the **Kleinert** program, the **Duran** program, and more recently a combination of the two, the **Washington** program (Dovelle & Heeter, 1989). The Kleinert program is probably the one that is used most frequently and is briefly described below.

## The Kleinert Program

The patient's wrist and hand are immobilized as follows:

- the wrist is 20° short of full flexion;
- the MPs are in 20° of flexion;
- the IPs are in 10° of flexion.

A dorsal back splint (Figure 4–10) is applied to maintain the fingers and wrist in the above positions. A rubber band extends from the dressing at the anterior aspect of the wrist to the fingernails and this is adjusted so that full active extension, within the confines of the dorsal back splint, is permitted. Once the extension is achieved the fingers return passively, because of the pull of the rubber band, to the palm of the hand. **There is no active contraction of the digital flexors during this exercise.** The patient performs this exercise as often as possible during the day for 3 weeks. The splint is removed at 3 weeks and a wrist band with

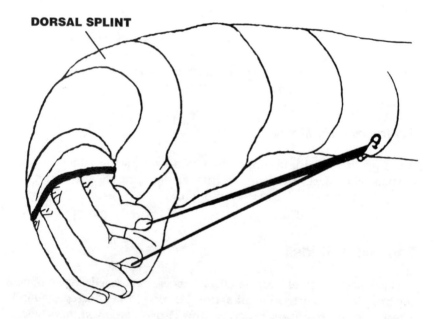

**DORSAL SPLINT**

**Figure 4–10.** Splinting of the hand following flexor tendon repair (adapted from Duran et al., 1984).

rubber band traction of the finger is fitted and the patient continues the exercises with the band in place for a further 3 weeks.

## SUMMARY

In this chapter common problems involving the elbow complex and selected conditions of the wrist and hand were discussed. It was also thought appropriate to include the Compartmental Syndrome in this chapter even though this condition is found in both the upper and lower extremities. The conditions relating to the elbow complex included Tennis Elbow and collateral Ligament Disorders.

The conditions selected for the wrist and hand were de Quervain's Disease, as an example of tenosynovitis, Carpal Tunnel Syndrome, as an example of an overuse injury, which involves the median nerve, Dupuytren's Disease involving the palmar fascia, Reflex Sympathetic Dystrophy of the hand as an example of a disorder of the autonomic nervous system and finally, as an example of the injured hand, a flexor tendon injury was selected.

# CHAPTER 5

# Thoracic, Lumbar, and Sacral Spines

Because of its length and growth changes, the thoracic spine is subject to postural deformity. The lumbosacral or weight bearing part of the spine is subject to stress trauma and resultant pain. Disc lesions in this region are very common as are associated problems of the zygapophyseal joints. The sacroiliac joint can be a source of discomfort as a result of biomechanical abnormalities.

## THE THORACIC SPINE

The chest cage and thoracic spine provide protection for the heart and lungs, but if deformed can compromise their function. The main focus of this section is on postural disorders that may occur in the thoracic spine.

## SCOLIOSIS

Scoliosis is a deformity resulting in a lateral curvature of the spine. It may be present as a **single curve** in the thoracic or lumbar region and sometimes in both; or it may present as a **double curve** with a lateral curvature in the thoracic spine and one in the lumbar region curving in the opposite direction. The curves commonly appear during adolescence when there is a spurt in growth, but they can appear in childhood (Koop, 1988).

A scoliosis is always described in terms of the **convexity** of the curve. One of the most common curve patterns is a right thoracic scoliosis which indicates that the convexity of the curve is to the right and the concavity is to the left. Often a compensatory curve is present in the opposite direction; for instance a left lumbar curve might be present as the compensatory curve for a right thoracic scoliosis. The right thoracic scoliosis would be termed the **major or primary** curve and the left lumbar curve would be called the **minor or secondary** curve.

## Classification

Scoliosis may be broadly classified under the two headings of non-structural scoliosis, which is reversible, and structural scoliosis, which is not reversible.

### Non-structural

The non-structural type of scoliosis results from one of the following **correctible** causes:

- habitual poor posture;
- lower limb length discrepancy, either because of an actual shortening, or because of tight musculature producing an apparent shortening of one leg; in both instances there is a tilt of the pelvis causing a lateral curvature in the lumbar region;
- pain, caused by a lumbar disc disorder or an abdominal problem such as a perinephric abscess, which will cause the patient to lean towards one side producing a lateral curvature.

### Structural

In structural scoliosis the lateral curvature is much more difficult to treat because of muscle contractures and bony changes and the curve **may be considered irreversible**; the category may be subdivided further as follows.

**Idiopathic.** This is of unknown origin but an abnormal growth pattern is present; it comprises about 85 percent of the structural type of scoliosis; it may be subdivided by age grouping:

- infantile—under 3 years of age;
- juvenile—age 3 to onset of puberty, usually age 9;
- adolescent—after age 10 until maturity.

**Osteopathic.** This type of scoliosis can be congenital and develop as a result of some defect in the spine, for example, a hemivertebra or a congenital fusion of the ribs. It can also be acquired and develop as a result of, for instance, fractures.

**Myopathic.** Scoliosis of this type affects the muscular development and is usually congenital, as in amyotonia congenita or muscular dystrophy.

**Neuropathic.** Scoliosis that is neuropathic in origin can be acquired, for instance as a result of poliomyelitis, or it can be congenital as in cerebral palsy.

Since idiopathic scoliosis is the most common type of structural scoliosis, it will serve as the focus of study of this complex condition.

# IDIOPATHIC SCOLIOSIS

The deformity of idiopathic scoliosis is **complex and progressive**. In addition to the clearly defined lateral flexion, there are areas of lordosis, kyphosis, rotation, and derotation; all of these may compromise cardiopulmonary function.

## Common Curve Patterns

There are four different curve patterns and these are described below.

### 1. Right Thoracic Curve

Right thoracic pattern is the most common pattern and commences at the fourth, fifth, or sixth thoracic vertebra and terminates at the eleventh or twelfth thoracic or at the first lumbar vertebra. It is always a major curve, and is structural. Smaller compensatory curves above or below the major curve are usually non-structural; they can become structural if present for a long time.

### 2. Thoracolumbar Curve

Thoracolumbar curve is fairly common. It is described as a long "C" curve and is usually to the right. It begins at the level of the fourth, fifth, or sixth thoracic vertebra and terminates at the level of the second, third, or fourth lumbar vertebra.

### 3. Right Thoracic and Left Lumbar Curve

Right thoracic and left lumbar is a double major curve which extends from the level of the fifth thoracic vertebra to the eleventh and from the eleventh thoracic vertebra to the fourth or fifth lumbar vertebra.

### 4. Left Lumbar Curve

The extent of left lumbar curve is from the eleventh or twelfth thoracic vertebra to the fifth lumbar vertebra.

## Measuring and Monitoring the Curve: The Cobb Method

Although there is more than one way of measuring and monitoring a curve the Cobb method (Figure 5–1) is the most widely used (Turek, 1984).

In this method the upper and lower end vertebrae are determined. These are the uppermost and lowermost vertebrae to tilt towards the concavity of the curve. The superior end vertebra is the **uppermost one in the curve whose superior surface points to the concavity** and the lower end vertebra is the one whose **inferior surface is the last one to point to the concavity of the curve**. Two horizontal lines are drawn, one parallel to the superior surface of the uppermost end vertebra and one parallel to the inferior surface of the lower end vertebra. Perpendiculars are drawn from these horizontal lines to intersect and the angle of intersection is considered the angle of the apex of the curve.

## Measuring and Monitoring the Rotation: X-Ray

The degree of rotation in a scoliosis is determined by the degree of rotation of the pedicle as seen on X-ray. A slight movement of the pedicle on the convex side backwards towards the midline would be described as a 1+. If the degree of rotation is such that only one vertebral pedicle is visible instead of two then the rotation is described as a 3+.

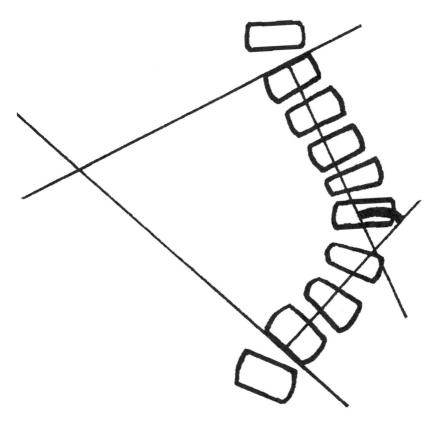

**Figure 5–1.** The Cobb method of measuring the degrees of deviation in idiopathic scoliosis (adapted from Turek, 1984).

## Progression of the Deformity

Double curves are likely to progress more rapidly than single curves and a single thoracic curve will progress more rapidly than a single lumbar curve (Lonstein,1988). Generally scoliosis ceases to progress significantly when a child reaches maturity. Girls reach maturity at about 16 years of age and boys at about 18. With this knowledge in mind it is possible to predict the curve's progression and consequently termination of treatment. Utilizing X-rays the apophyses of the iliac crests are studied. Their osseous centers start forming laterally and progress medially towards the sacrum. When the ilia are firmly sealed to the sacrum, maturation becomes complete and treatment can be discontinued.

## Anatomical Changes

The significant anatomical changes relate to the vertebrae and the rib cage.

### The Vertebrae

The bodies of the vertebrae rotate toward the convex side and the spinous processes toward the concave side. There is a decrease in vertebral and disc height on the concave side.

### The Rib Cage

As a result of the rotation of the vertebrae the ribs approximate each other on the concave side and are wider apart than normal on the convex side. In addition the ribs are pushed posteriorly on the convex side producing a visible rib **hump** and are pushed anteriorly on the concave side. Sometimes an anterior hump is present on the concave side.

## Differentiation Between the Structural and Non-Structural Curve

The lateral curve is visible when the patient is in the standing position in both structural and non-structural curves. When the patient is asked to bend forward to touch the toes the lateral curve and posterior hump will still be visible if they are caused by structural scoliosis, but will disappear if the curve is non-structural.

When traction is applied to the spine the structural or major curve remains, but the compensatory or minor curve will straighten out. The same thing occurs on side bending, but this is seen better on X-ray.

## Complications of Structural Scoliosis

With the advent of a structural scoliotic deformity deterioration in cardiorespiratory efficiency occurs; abnormal functional changes occur in involved muscles and there are associated pain patterns.

## Cardiorespiratory Insufficiency

The major complication in structural scoliosis is cardiorespiratory insufficiency. This seldom appears with curves of less than 65°. Right thoracic curves in particular tend to cause cardiorespiratory problems, because of narrowing of the chest cavity which limits heart function as well as lung expansion.

### Abnormal Functioning of Muscles

In severe deformities the direction of the fibers of certain muscles becomes so altered that their function changes. Because of this changed function the muscles may well contribute to the progression of the deformity.

### Associated Pain and Muscle Ache

Winter, Lonstein, and Denis (1988) have identified several pain patterns found in patients with scoliosis. However, they point out that careful assessment and analysis are necessary in order to determine that the cause of the patient's pain is attributable to the scoliosis and not to some unassociated musculoskeletal disorder. van Dam, Bradford, Lonstein, Moe, Ogilvie, and Winter (1987) identify pain as the main factor for surgical intervention in the adult patient with idiopathic scoliosis.

## Clinical Examination

Early detection of the idiopathic scoliosis facilitates treatment and the following aspects of the clinical examination are carried out carefully.

### Screening

Scoliosis in its early stages is frequently not apparent to the untrained eye. It is the responsibility of physical therapists and other professionals to carefully examine all the children they are treating for evidence of structural scoliosis. The sooner treatment begins the better is the chance of controlling the deformity.

## Observation

The symmetry of the levels of the ears, shoulders, inferior angles of the scapulae, iliac crests, and knee creases must be checked from the posterior aspect. A right thoracic scoliosis should be suspected if the shoulder and inferior angle of the scapula are higher on the right side.

Note should be made of skin tumors and of any markings on the skin, such as "cafe au lait" spots. The presence of these are signs of neurofibromatosis, which is one of the neuropathic causes of scoliosis. The presence of hair in the lumbar region may indicate the presence of spina bifida which is another neuropathic cause of scoliosis.

## Mobility Tests and Measurements

It is important to perform mobility tests and to take specific measurements when monitoring the progress of the condition. The physical therapist should monitor postural and functional changes.

**Flexibility of Rib Cage and Spine.** It is important to test and monitor flexibility in the forward flexed position to determine whether or not the rib hump disappears. Lifting the child up by supporting under both sides of the mandible will also stretch the spine; the scoliosis will disappear if it is non-structural.

**Mobility of Chest Cage in Respiration.** The mobility of the chest cage is an important factor in scoliosis as it affects maximum breathing capacity. The range of movement and the vital capacity should both be monitored.

**Limb Length Discrepancy (LLD).** An anatomical shortness of one limb can produce in standing a lateral tilt of the pelvis with a compensatory scoliosis. The extent of the shortness can be determined by placing blocks 1/16 of an inch thick beneath the short limb until the posterior iliac spines are equal (Subotnick, 1981).

**Balanced Spine.** A balanced spine has a better prognosis than an unbalanced one. It can be identified by dropping a plumb line from the spinous process of the seventh cervical vertebra and noting if it is in line with the gluteal cleft.

## Conservative Management

### Braces

The Milwaukee brace (Blount & Moe, 1980) is a longstanding success story in the treatment of idiopathic scoliosis with up to a 40° curvature, since it first appeared in 1945. This is particularly so of right thoracic curves with some flexibility. It has been used with exercises in and out of the brace. Because of the poor compliance of the patient regarding the exercises and lack of supporting evidence as to their value the specific exercise program has been replaced by a general exercise and activity program in some instances (Lonstein & Winter, 1988).

Another type of brace which is proving effective is the underarm brace. This either extends up to one or both axillae and is known as the higher brace, or does not extend as high as the axillae and is known as the lower brace. The higher brace is used for the thoracic curve and the lower brace for the thoraco-lumbar and lumbar curves (Lonstein & Winter, 1988).

### Lateral Electrical Surface Stimulation (LESS)

This approach to treatment was first introduced by McCullough (1986) in 1971. Electrodes are applied to the surface on the convex side of the curve and are used only at night. Treatment is continued until the end of growth. This approach to treatment is suitable for curves up to 39°.

Other conservative approaches to treatment involve traction and casting.

## Surgical Instrumentation

The **Harrington rod instrumentation** and spinal fusion for treatment of idiopathic scoliosis has been the most successful surgical means of correction for many years for curves extending from the upper thoracic region to the level of the fourth lumbar vertebra. The early stage of this procedure involves the introduction of the "outrigger" to elongate the spine on the concave side of the curve (Figure 5–2). The elongation is then maintained by inserting a distraction rod to replace the "outrigger." A major drawback was lengthy immobilization for 4, 6, or 8 months, depending on the circumstances, in a synthetic cast to ensure stability. Also the instrumentation had limited derotation and sagittal plane control.

The addition of **transverse traction devices** that anchor the distraction rod to a compression rod has, in recent years, increased the stability of the Harrington instrumentation.

The introduction of **Luque wiring** (segmental lateral correc-

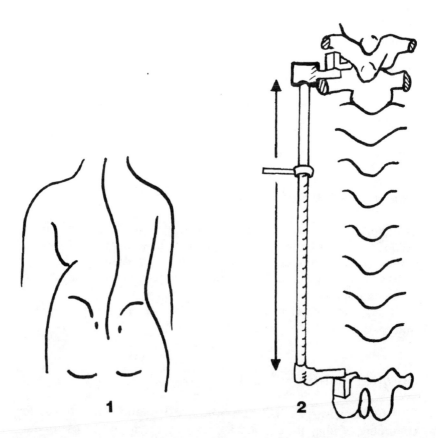

**Figure 5–2.**   (1) Right thoracic scoliosis and (2) the Harrington outrigger in place (adapted from Turek, 1984).

tion and fixation utilizing sublaminar wiring) with Harrington instrumentation went a step further and produced a system far stronger than the Harrington rod, either by itself or combined with a compression rod (Silverman & Greenbarg, 1988). It also had the advantage of increasing the sagittal plane control. However, a brace must be worn for three months postoperatively.

The **Cotrel-Dubousset instrumentation** provides sufficient stability to allow the patient to go without a brace postoperatively. This system consists of two rods, which are placed on either side of the posterior elements, and attached to the spine by multiple hooks. Two devices for transverse traction crosslink the two rods (Denis, 1988). This system has yet to stand the test of time and so far the rate of complication has been higher than in the Harrington instrumentation.

Generally speaking, instrumentation is suitable for a skeletally immature patient with a curve of 40° and above. Curves below this range are treated conservatively.

## OSTEOPOROSIS

In the individual with osteoporosis the bone tissue is reduced in comparison with others of the same age and sex (Courpron, 1981). Loss of bone mass is part of the aging process; osteoporosis develops when the rate of bone formation is exceeded by the rate of bone absorption. However, it has been reported that less than a third of the population develops osteoporosis (Kleerekoper, Tolia, & Parfitt, 1981). Women are affected more than men. Although osteoporosis is a generalized condition the most dramatic changes occur in the spine and particularly the thoracic spine. The vertebrae become wedge shaped anteriorly as a result of the excessive bone absorption and compression forces. Thoracic kyphosis is evident, and fractures develop, often from trivial activities (Turek, 1984).

### Etiology

The following factors are considered to be influential in the development of osteoporosis:

- inadequate calcium metabolism;
- protein deficiency possibly caused by gastrointestinal disturbances;
- hormonal disturbances, particularly resulting in a loss of estrogen associated with the post-menopause phase;

- inactivity, particularly prolonged immobilization;
- vitamin D deficiency;
- long term use of corticosteroids.

## Treatment Guidelines

Medical treatment may include estrogen therapy, administration of calcium, vitamin D, and sodium fluoride.

From the viewpoint of physical therapy, thoracic extension exercises have been advocated (McKenzie, 1990; Turek, 1984). These may be performed in the sitting, supine, and prone lying positions (Aisenbrey, 1987). Activity, particularly in the weight bearing position, and general exercises are also helpful.

## DISC LESIONS

Mechanical problems in the thoracic spine are rare. Kramer (1981) has shown that only 1.96 percent of patients with back pain have a mechanical disorder of the thoracic spine. McKenzie (1990) has identified posterior and posterolateral derangements caused by disc lesions, but he, too, reports that they are rare.

## Clinical Features

Central or symmetrical pain adjacent to the midline between the first and the twelfth thoracic vertebrae, with or without radiating pain around the chest wall, is indicative of such a disc lesion.

## Treatment Guidelines

The extension approach to treatment as described by McKenzie (1990) in prone lying is implemented. If this approach is ineffective, extension and rotation mobilizations are performed.

*Note:* The above treatment approaches are the same as those used for derangements in the lumbar region. These are described in detail in the next chapter.

# THE LUMBAR AND SACRAL SPINES

Disorders in the lumbar and sacral regions usually result in the common condition known as "low back pain."

The number of people who experience low back pain far exceeds those suffering from any other form of joint pain. The loss in labor hours and the cost in terms of compensation and medical care for the treatment of this problem have been astronomical. According to Anderson (1987) 60,000,000 work days are lost each year in the United States and another 15,000,000 in Britain as a result of back pain. The remainder of this chapter examines the anatomical structures implicated in this costly disorder, as well as the more common conditions responsible for it.

## PERTINENT ANATOMICAL ASPECTS

The region of the back which is affected the most by disc lesions is the lumbar spine, and the causative structure is commonly a component of the three-joint complex involving the intervertebral disc and the two zygapophyseal joints and related ligaments (Figure 5–3). Although there are obvious anatomical differences between the cervical and the lumbar spines, such as function, size, and shape of the IVF, vertebral canal and vertebrae, orientation of the facets, and direction of the nerve roots, there are many similarities in terms of the pathology of the three-joint complex. For a comprehensive description of this joint complex refer to Chapter 2.

It is obvious that the large lumbar vertebral body is designed for weightbearing. However, it has been estimated that, in the erect position, 15 per cent of the superincumbent weight is borne by the zygapophyseal joints (Adams & Hutton, 1980), and that with increased lordosis this weightbearing percentage is increased. The increased size of the transverse and spinous processes provides an anchorage for the strong back muscles. The orientation of the articular surfaces of the zygapophyseal joints provides a means of restraining certain movements: since this orientation varies in different parts of the lumbar spine it is worthy of some discussion.

## The Zygapophyseal Joints

The zygapophyseal joints are synovial joints formed by the articulation between the superior surfaces of one vertebra with the inferior surfaces of the vertebra above; they are also known as "facet" or "posterior" joints.

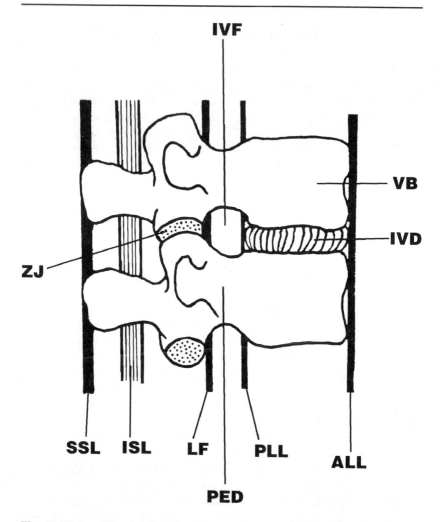

**Figure 5–3.** The lumbar functional unit and ligamentous structures. Intervertebral foramen (IVF), vertebral body (VB), intervertebral disc (IVD), anterior longitudinal ligament (ALL), posterior longitudinal ligament (PLL), pedicle (PED), ligamentum flavum (LF), interspinous ligament (ISL), supraspinous ligament (SSL), and zygapophyseal joint (ZJ) (adapted from Cailliet, 1988).

## Orientation of the Articulating Surfaces

The orientation of the articular surfaces varies from an oblique or curved orientation to a flat orientation; the former is more prevalent in the upper lumbar region and the latter is more prevalent at L4-L5 and L5-S1. This orientation has an effect on the movements produced in the different parts of the lumbar spine (Bogduk & Twomey, 1991).

### Effects of Certain Movements

On forward flexion the inferior articular surfaces ride upward on the superior articular surfaces of the vertebra below, causing stretching of the posterior soft tissue structures and compression of the anterior soft tissue structures. The reverse happens in extension.

On lateral flexion to the left, the right inferior articular surface rides upward on the right superior articular surface, thus stretching the soft tissue structures on the right side and compressing those on the left. The reverse happens with right lateral flexion.

If forward flexion and left lateral flexion are combined the stretching effects on the right are increased, and there is slight stretching of the structures on the left. Similarly, if extension is combined with left side flexion there is an increase in the compression force on the left and a decrease on the right (Edwards, 1987). These combined movements are used in both assessment and treatment (Edwards, 1987; Trott, Grant, & Maitland, 1987).

# DCSIONS

Intervertebral discs have been implicated as a major causative factor in low back pain (Cyriax, 1982; McKenzie, 1981; Mooney, 1987).

# Pathology

The types of disc disturbances that appear to cause the most severe symptoms are those in which the disc material moves in a posterior or posterolateral direction (Figure 5–4). The disc may impinge on nerve root, spinal ligaments, or spinal cord, giving rise to pain and limitation of movements. The less common anterior protrusion may stress the anterior longitudinal ligament and thus limit spinal flexion. Protrusion of disc material in a caudal or cephalic direction through a gap in the endplate is a very common occurrence. Such protrusions enter the vertebral body and are often of very small diameter and symptomless; they are called Schmorl's nodes (Vernon-Roberts, 1987).

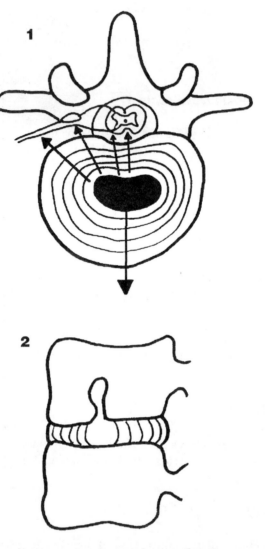

**Figure 5–4.** Direction of lumbar disc lesions: (1) posterior, posterolateral and anterior; and (2) into the body of the vertebra (Schmorl's node).

Macnab (1977) has made the following differentiation between disc protrusion and herniation (Figure 5–5).

### Disc Protrusion

The fibers of the annulus fibrosus remain intact, but as degeneration occurs and the disc decreases in size the annulus bulges either

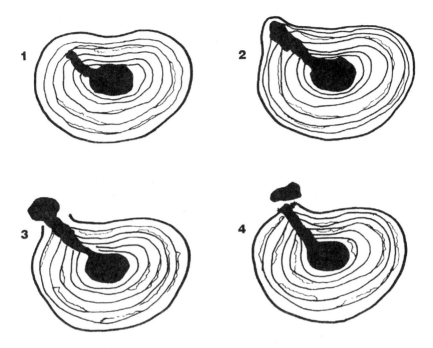

**Figure 5–5.** Types of lumbar disc lesions: (1) leakage of nuclear material through the inner rings of the annulus fibrosus; (2) protrusion; (3) herniation; and (4) sequestration (adapted from Macnab, 1977).

locally or generally. If the latter occurs the annulus forms a bulging rim between the vertebral bodies.

### Disc Herniations

Disc herniations consist of three types and in each type **disruption** of the annular fibers has occurred.

**Prolapsed Intervertebral Disc.** There is a local prominence of the annulus which contains a few fibers only. When these are torn the nucleus will ooze out (see below).

**Extruded Intervertebral Disc.** Nucleus material oozes through the damaged fibers of the annulus and comes to rest beneath the posterior longitudinal ligament.

**Sequestrated Intervertebral Disc.**  Nuclear material oozes through the annulus and the posterior longitudinal ligament, breaks away, and may rest in the spinal canal or more commonly, in the intervertebral foramen (IVF).

## Common Sites

Disc lesions at the fourth and fifth lumbar joints are the most common and the fourth and fifth lumbar roots are the ones which are most often affected. According to Cyriax (1982) evidence of a fourth lumbar root involvement is indicative of a lesion at the fourth joint level. However, as he has found, a disc lesion at the fourth joint level can equally compress the fifth nerve root, and the first and second sacral nerve roots can be compressed by a fifth lumbar disc protrusion; this should be borne in mind when directing treatment by manual therapy at specific joint levels.

The full root syndromes described below include pain and other sensory changes which may be referred to the appropriate dermatome (Figure 5–6), and neural deficits such as muscle weakness; however, it must be remembered that the full root syndrome is not always present. When it is, treatment by mechanical means is not as effective as when neural deficits are not present (Cyriax, 1982; McKenzie, 1981).

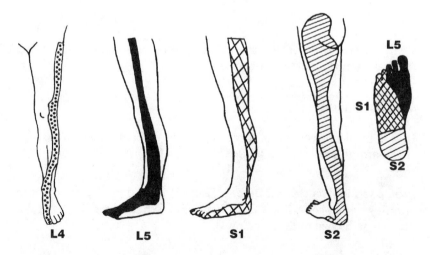

**Figure 5–6.**   Dermatomes of the lower extremity L4 to S2.

## Mechanism of Injury

Severe back pain often develops suddenly when the patient is in the flexed position; she or he is unable to regain the erect position because of pain and locking of the joint. However, degeneration of the disc has occurred prior to the painful onset. These degenerative processes make the disc more vulnerable to sudden movements and sustained stresses.

## Clinical Features

The following clinical features assist the therapist in identifying the level at which the lesion is occurring.

### Fourth Lumbar (L4) Root

The fourth lumbar nerve root is most commonly subjected to compression.

- Pain is experienced in the mid lumbar region or in the iliac crest.
- A lateral deviation of the lumbar curve is present.
- There is limitation of side flexion unilaterally, or a painful arc in side flexion may be present in less severe lesions.
- Referred pain is experienced in the fourth lumbar (L4) dermatome, more often distally than proximally.
- There is a positive response to the straight leg raising test (SLR) which may be unilateral or bilateral and is increased on neck flexion.
- Numbness is present in the outer part of the leg or the great toe.
- Weakness of tibialis anterior and extensor hallucis longus may be present.

### Fifth Lumbar (L5) Root

Disc lesions at the fifth lumbar joint are almost as common as those at the fourth joint level.

- Lateral deviation (Figure 5–7) may be seen either towards, or, more commonly,away from the painful side, or lateral deviation may occur only on forward flexion.
- The partial articular pattern is present—some movements are restricted, others are not.

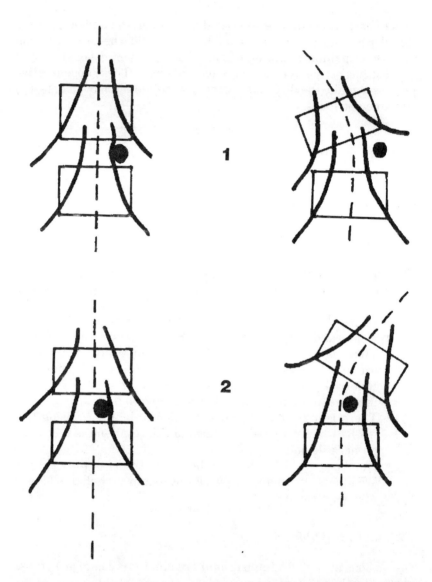

**Figure 5–7.** Lateral deviation of the spine in relation to the location of the disc lesion: (1) lesion located lateral to the nerve root, the patient leans away from the protrusion; (2) lesion located medial to the nerve root, the patient leans toward the protrusion (adapted form Kirkaldy-Willis, 1983).

- There is a positive response to SLR which is increased on neck flexion.
- Pain is experienced in the fifth lumbar (L5) dermatome more often distally than proximally.
- Numbness of the outer leg and inner three toes is present.
- Weakness is evident in gluteus medius, peronei, and extensor hallucis longus.
- There is a sluggish or absent ankle reflex (Cyriax, 1982).

### First Sacral (S1) and Second Sacral (S2) Roots

As stated previously, the S1 and S2 roots can be compressed by a disc lesion at the fifth lumbar joint level.

- Pain is experienced in the respective dermatomes.
- There is weakness of the hamstring and calf muscles; the peronei are also weak in the S1 nerve root involvement.
- Numbness may be experienced in the lower part of the outer leg, outer foot, and the lateral two toes with an S1 problem, and down the posterior aspect of the limb and in to the heel with S2 involvement.
- SLR is limited.

## Treatment Guidelines

White and Panjabi (1978) have identified a position which will help to relieve LBP (Figure 5–8), particularly if the LBP is associated with a disc lesion. It is effective because disc pressure is reduced in the supine position; tension is removed from the sciatic nerve and the iliopsoas muscle when the hips and knees are flexed, and the straight back helps to contain bulging of the disc posteriorly.

The disc lesions which do not involve neural deficits such as muscular weakness respond well to manual techniques involving extension and rotation. These have been well described by Cyriax (1984), Maitland (1986), and McKenzie (1981). The approaches may differ in technique but the principles involved are similar. A "hands off" approach involving extension is described in the next chapter.

## Cauda Equina Lesion

In the presence of a large posterior protrusion the posterior longitudinal ligament will rupture and the disc will exert pressure on the cauda equina. The sciatic nerve roots on both sides are compressed.

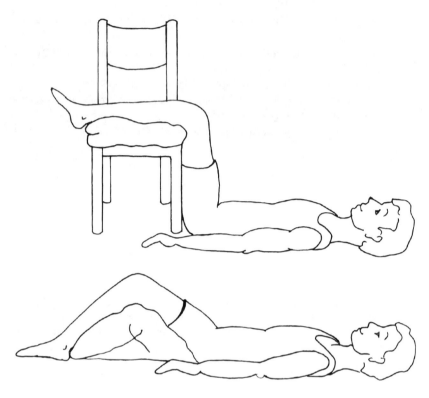

**Figure 5–8.** Positions of comfort for low back pain (adapted from White & Panjabi, 1978).

## Clinical Features

- Pressure on the third and fourth sacral roots causes weakness of the bladder and may cause permanent paralysis.
- Bilateral sciatica is present along with lower sacral and perineal pain.
- There is bilateral limitation of straight-leg raising.
- Analgesia of the saddle area, perineum, and anus is present.
- There is weakness of the anal and bladder sphincters.

*Note:* Severe disc problems may warrant a period of bed rest prior to treatment by physical means.

## LUMBAR SPONDYLOSIS

In Chapter 2 the three-joint complex and its inter-relationships were described in detail. The same relationship exists in the lumbar spine, in that if the intervertebral joint is not functioning properly it will have adverse effects on the function of the zygapophyseal joints and vice versa. The lowest two levels are affected the most, probably because they are the transition levels to a more rigid structure—the sacrum. The degenerative changes of lumbar spondylosis in the three-joint complex are responsible for disc lesions, degeneration in the zygapophyseal joints, degenerative spondylolisthesis, and spinal stenosis (Figure 5–9).

The following is a brief interpretation of the process of degeneration in the lumbar spine as described by Yong-Hing & Kirkaldy-Willis (1983).

The first stage in the degenerative disease process is one of **dysfunction** where there are minor pathological changes resulting in some loss of joint movement; these changes are reversible. If the disease progresses it moves into the second stage, that of **instability**; finally there is the stage of **stabilization**.

### Dysfunction

Small degenerative changes in the disc and minor capsular tears cause some degree of subluxation in the zygapophyseal joints resulting in synovitis. Muscle spasm develops in order to protect the joint from adverse movement. The sustained muscle contraction causes ischemia and resultant pain, which may be local or referred; movements are restricted.

### Instability

In the first stage the problem was almost entirely localized to the zygapophyseal joints. With the onset of the unstable stage further stresses have adverse effects on the zygapophyseal joints—degeneration of the cartilage, and stretching and laxity of the capsule. The disc undergoes further degenerative changes resulting in protrusion of the annulus. The effects of the degenerative stages taking place in the three-joint complex cause an increase in abnormal movement resulting in instability.

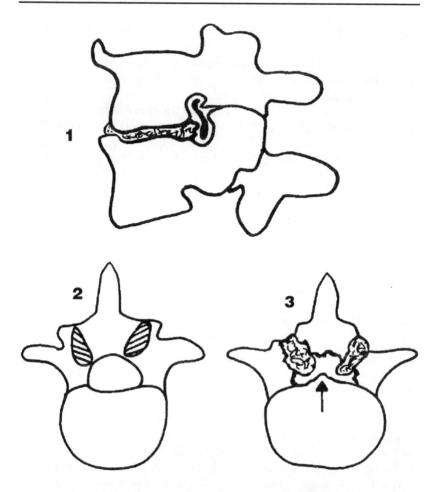

**Figure 5–9.** (1) Lumbar spondylosis and resultant degenerative changes. (2) Normal configuration of the spinal canal. (3) Spinal stenosis as a result of the degenerative process involving the disc and zygapophyseal joints (2 & 3 adapted from Arhrnoldi et al., 1976).

The symptoms associated with this stage in the degenerative process are a progression of those experienced in the stage of dysfunction—the pain is more frequent and increased in intensity, and there is a feeling of weakness in the back.

## Stabilization

In stabilization, the final stage, movement is restricted in the zygapophyseal joints because of advanced degenerative changes resulting in fibrosis of the zygapophyseal joints, an increase in size, and locking of the articular surfaces. Similar degenerative changes occur in the disc, resulting in loss of disc space and osteophyte formation. The painful symptoms decrease in intensity and the patient, on the whole, is able to function with much less discomfort, albeit with a limited range of motion.

*Note:* The above three stages have been described separately but they do overlap and although they usually develop in one segment only, they later spread to other segments. Nerve root compression can occur in the lateral nerve root canal either during the late stage of stage two (instability) or in stage three (stabilization).

## STENOSIS

In stenosis there is a narrowing of one or all of the following canals or apertures (Kirkaldy-Willis & McIvor, 1976):

- the **spinal or vertebral canal** which runs vertically behind the vertebral bodies and houses the spinal cord;
- the **nerve root canal** which extends from the point where the nerve root sheath comes off the dural sac, and terminates where the nerve root emerges from the intervertebral foramen;
- the **intervertebral foramen** which is bounded anteriorly by the vertebral bodies and discs and posteriorly by the ligamentum flavum, the pars interarticularis, and the upper portion of the superior facet; the roof and floor are formed by the pedicles (Figure 5–3).

The condition may be local or generalized in the lumbar spine; the stenosis or narrowing of one or all of the above canals and apertures may be caused by bone or soft tissue invasion. A combination of factors may exist, for instance a congenitally small spinal canal plus osteophytic invasion from the facet joints, or disc herniation in the presence of degeneration of the facet joints. The result is nerve root entrapment and probably vascular compression.

## Clinical Features

The clinical features of spinal stenosis and disc herniation are similar. It therefore seems appropriate to make distinctions between the two conditions.

### Spinal Stenosis

The mean age of onset is the latter part of the fourth decade and over.

Back pain is present for some time before the patient's leg pain appears; the back pain is not acute.

Painful stiffness develops with inactivity, which the patient eases in 2–3 hours with activity.

Nerve root pain is not specific in its localization.

Bilateral leg pains are common.

The patient suffers few acute attacks, but has a more grumbling type of pain in the back and legs that persists over a long period of time and tends to become progressively worse.

Symptoms of intermittent neurogenic claudication of the cauda equina in both legs may appear with walking and disappear with rest and spinal flexion.

Spinal movements are not as restricted as in disc herniation.

SLR is not as restricted as with a disc herniation.

Sitting often relieves the pain because space in the spinal canal is increased.

Decreasing ability to walk is evident over a period of 2 years.

### Disc Herniation

The mean age of onset is the early part of the fourth decade

Leg pain appears fairly soon after the onset of back pain; the back pain is usually acute.

Pain tends to develop with activity and ease with rest.

Nerve root pain is acute and specific in its localization.

Bilateral leg pain is uncommon.

The patient has recurrent attacks of pain that may be severe, but clear with conservative treatment.

Intermittent neurogenic claudication of the cauda equina is uncommon.

Spinal movements are more restricted than in spinal stenosis.

SLR is more restricted than in stenosis.

Sitting increases pain because of the increase in intradiscal pressure in the sitting position.

The patient may be unable to walk, usually because of acute pain.

Walking uphill (spine in flexion) is easier than walking downhill (spine in extension).

Patients with neurogenic claudication adopt a posture of flexed hips and knees (Porter, 1987).

## Treatment Guidelines

It becomes obvious from the above observations that the patient with spinal stenosis is more comfortable in the flexed than in the extended position, because the canals are enlarged, thus providing more space for contained structures (Wiltse, Kirkaldy-Willis, & McIvor, 1976). Porter (1987) cites the cycle test as a means of distinguishing between intermittent claudication that occurs in peripheral vascular disease, and neurogenic claudication. In intermittent claudication the distance the patient is able to cycle is the same whether the spine is flexed or extended. In neurogenic claudication the distance is decreased when the spine is extended.

### *Conservative*

Back education and exercises are focused upon maintaining a flexed rather than a lordotic position of the spine. However, it must be remembered that conservative treatment is of limited value.

### *Surgical*

A decompression procedure may be performed.

## SPONDYLOLYSIS

This condition most commonly affects the fifth lumbar vertebra and less frequently the fourth lumbar vertebra. It is attributable to a defect in the pars interarticularis (the part of the lamina between the inferior and superior facets). It is present in 10 per cent of adults (Salter, 1983).

## Etiology

It has been suggested that spondylolysis is probably caused by a stress fracture in the pars interarticularis that fails to heal properly (Salter, 1983; Troup, 1976), or of both the pars interarticularis and the pedicle (Lamy, Bazergui, Kraus, & Farfan, 1975). Ahead of the defect lies the superior facet and the vertebral body; behind the defect are the inferior facet and spinous process (Figure 5–10). The condition itself need not give rise to symptoms, but the segment may be unstable and the pars interarticularis is vulnerable. This is particularly so in the presence of an increase in lordosis of the lumbar spine (Adams & Hutton, 1980), which results in greater stresses on the vertebral arch (Ogilvie & Sherman, 1987). If the defect is present bilaterally, elongation or separation can occur and the condition leads to spondylolisthesis.

## SPONDYLOLISTHESIS

Spondylolisthesis is the sliding of one vertebra on another, usually occurring at L5-S1 and less commonly at L4-L5. Under normal circumstances this sliding forward is prevented by the vertebral arch and the posterior facets (Ogilvie & Sherman, 1987). The condition has been described by Mooney (1983) as a source of segmental instability, the severity of which is determined by the degree of slip of the upper vertebra on the lower one. In most instances the condition develops as a result of spondylolysis as described above, or less commonly because of congenital defects in the facets (Adams & Hamblen, 1990; Macnab, 1977). The slide is in an anterior direction. At the L5-S1 level the L5 vertebral body and the superior facet will slide forward and downward on S1 carrying with it the vertebrae above. The spinous process and inferior facet remain behind (Figure 5–10). The slide forward may be slight, asymptomatic, and may or may not be detectable by X-ray. A slip of one half the depth of the vertebral body is serious, because the sciatic nerve roots will be stretched and the condition will require surgical intervention in the form of a fusion.

## Clinical Features

As indicated earlier the condition in its mildest form can be asymptomatic; the following features are present in the more advanced stage of the disorder.

- Backache may be evident, particularly after activity.
- Nerve root signs in both legs may be present in advanced cases because of traction of the nerve roots.

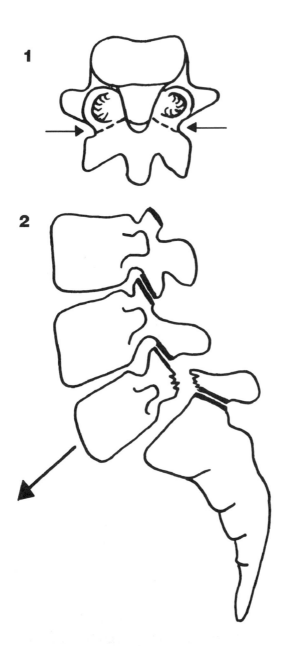

**Figure 5–10.** (1) Spondylolisis with the defect in the pars interarticularis. (2) Spondylolisthesis of the fifth vertebra (adapted from Moore, 1980).

- The buttocks appear flat.
- A "step" is felt at the level below where the listhesis has occurred.
- Transverse creases appear in the region of the waist.
- The abdomen is protruding.

## Treatment Guidelines

### Conservative

The slip of the vertebra is encouraged by the lumbosacral angle and the pull of gravity; consequently, the focus of conservative treatment is on counteracting these adverse forces. Such a program would include the following:

- lifting techniques and postural education;
- pelvic tilting and abdominal strengthening to counteract the lordotic posture.

*Note:* In a limited study carried out by Gramse, Sinaki, and Ilstrup (1980), the above conservative approach to treatment was found to be beneficial, whereas extension exercises increased the patient's pain.

### Surgical Intervention

Surgery involves fusion of the involved segments.

## ZYGAPOPHYSEAL JOINT SYNDROMES

As will be seen later there is an element of controversy relating to zygapophyseal syndromes. Although referred pain is not a clinical feature in the syndromes described below it can develop, and it is this feature which is the probable cause of the controversy (see Note below at the end of the section on zygapophyseal joint syndromes).

## A. SPRAIN

The zygapophyseal joint on one side can be sprained by a minor movement involving flexion to the opposite side (Macnab, 1977) or by moderate to severe trauma (Saunders, 1979). In both mechanisms the capsule of the joint is injured.

## Clinical Features

The patient presents with the following signs and symptoms:

- severe incapacitating pain;
- inability to move because of rigid splinting of the lumbar spine by muscle spasm;
- slight flexion of the hips and knees in walking (Porter, 1987).

## Conservative Treatment Guidelines

The approach is the same as for other joint sprains:

- bed rest (if practical) with physical therapy modalities during the acute stage;
- gentle pain free movements to prevent loss of movement in the joint;
- progression to full range movements and normal strength when healing has taken place.

## B. LOCKING

Rahlmann (1987) identifies meniscoid entrapment, displaced intervertebral disc fragments, muscle spasm, and periarticular connective tissue adhesions as possible causes of intervertebral joint fixation (joint locking). The use of the word "locking" to describe this condition is open to debate and perhaps "meniscoid entrapment" as described by Bogduk and Twomey (1991) is more appropriate.

## Mechanism of Injury

The patient moves quickly into forward flexion and as he or she does so a fibrous adipose meniscus is drawn out of the joint; this meniscus fails to be reduced when the patient tries to extend. Instead of being restored to its normal position it impinges and blocks the joint.

## Clinical Features

The following features are present:

- the patient experiences severe pain in the back;
- there is an inability to move into extension because of the pain, and when the patient is able to do so the pain is localized lateral to the spinous process at a specific level;

## Conservative Treatment Guidelines

The condition responds well to a manipulation involving flexion and rotation.

*Note:* It is important to point out that several authorities, for instance Farfan (1973) and Bogduk and Twomey (1991), believe it is extremely difficult to isolate a problem with the zygapophyseal joint from a problem involving the intervertebral joint complex. Mooney and Robertson (1976) point out that when referred pain is a feature of a zygapophyseal disorder it cannot be differentiated from that associated with a disc problem. Diminished reflex activity and limitation of straight leg raising have also been found to be associated with zygapophyseal irritation.

## LUMBOSACRAL STRAIN

Because of the extreme angulation at this joint, it is vulnerable to extension stresses, which may lead to an acute or chronic disorder.

## A. ACUTE

In all probability lumbosacral sprain is caused by a posterior (zygapophyseal) joint strain superimposed on an unstable segment. With the advent of disc degeneration segmental instability develops; this makes the back vulnerable to unguarded movements such as posterior joint strain. Hyperextension may occur in the segments and if additional extension strains are imposed the joints are pushed beyond their physiological limits causing pain. Eventually subluxation of the zygapophyseal joints may occur.

## Treatment Guidelines

Treatment consists of:

- rest, anti-inflammatory drugs, sedatives;
- postural education, abdominal exercises.

## B. CHRONIC

Unlike the acute form, which can develop suddenly, the chronic form develops slowly. The entire process is aggravated further if the patient has excess weight in the abdominal region and weak abdominals; both lead to degenerative changes in the facet joints.

## Treatment Guidelines

Since the problem is essentially one of excessive lordosis or hyperextension, the treatment approach is to correct the postural problem. There will also be some loss of flexion present that will have to be restored.

- Diet is important to reduce the "paunch" and the stress on the joints.
- General education regarding posture, correct lifting techniques, posterior pelvic tilting, and movements into flexion are the principles of treatment.
- The height of the shoe heel is important, since high heels tend to encourage hyperextension.

## THE SACROILIAC JOINT (SIJ)

Problems in the lumbar region can refer pain to the SIJ which may even be tender on palpation. This phenomenon has misled practitioners in the past into believing that the SIJ is a common cause of pain in this region. Also asymmetry in the pelvic region became the focus of excessive attention which may or may not have been justified. However, there are syndromes associated with this joint that warrant attention.

The joint is extremely stable because of the bony architecture and strong ligamentous support. Its cartilaginous surfaces are well developed and it has a synovial membrane. There is an available range of 3–5° of rotation in the younger person, but after the fifth decade fibrosis takes place. The function of the joint is twofold:

- to serve as a buffer between the lumbosacral region and the hip joints;
- to provide the pelvic ring with some flexibility (Kirkaldy-Willis, 1983), especially in women during the childbearing years.

## Mechanism of Injury

Several mechanisms have been identified:

- a fall on the buttocks;
- severe trauma such as that sustained in a motor vehicle accident;
- stepping down unexpectedly from a deep step;
- sustained muscle contraction;
- childbirth.

## Clinical Features

Some of the clinical features are specific and others are not.

- There is pain over the SIJ and/or pubic symphysis.
- The pain may be referred in varying patterns, but a common pattern of referral is to the posterolateral buttock and over the greater trochanter to the anterior thigh.
- Most movements such as walking, climbing stairs, changing from standing to sitting and the reverse, will increase the discomfort.
- The patient may walk with a limp.

## Syndromes

Syndromes commonly relate to hypomobility of the the sacroiliac joint. Syndromes related to anterior or posterior rotation of the innominate bone can be myofascial or articular in origin and those related to superior subluxations (upslips), in either anterior or posterior rotation, are articular in origin.

In order to determine the cause of the patient's problem, careful examination of the bilateral relationships of the anterior superior iliac spines, the posterior iliac spines, and the ischial tuberosities is essential. In addition, the posteroanterior relationship of the right sacral base must be compared with that of the left sacral base and the posteroanterior relationships of both inferior lateral angles of the sacrum must be compared with each other. Finally, the two sacral sulci must be compared in terms of depth (Lee, 1989). In addition, all musculature that could influence the SIJ, such as those of the hip, must be examined for tightness and/or weakness.

## Treatment

Treatment involves release of associated tight musculature, passive mobilizations to restore normal alignment, followed by active exercises to maintain normal alignment and to prevent recurrence.

## NON-MUSCULOSKELETAL CAUSES OF LOW BACK PAIN

Macnab (1977) has established that back pain may develop from one or other of the following sources:

**1.** *Vascular.* A deep-seated lumbar pain that does not increase with activity nor decrease with rest could be an aortic aneurysm. The pulsations from the aneurysm can be felt in the abdomen and the aneurysm itself causes low back pain as a result of the pressure it exerts on sensitive structures.

A pain in the legs similar to sciatica is experienced in peripheral vascular disease. It causes limping and is brought on by walking. It is relieved by standing still. The condition is called "intermittent claudication."

**2.** *Neurological.* The most likely causes are cysts and tumors involving the nerve roots, such as neurolemmomata and neurofibromata. These are often difficult to distinguish from other nerve root problems such as compression. One clinical feature exhibited in cysts or tumors but absent in nerve root compression is the patient's report of having to get out of bed and walk around to ease the pain.

**3.** *Viscerogenic.* Disease of the kidneys or pelvic viscera may give rise to low back pain. However, low back pain from disease of the viscera will not change with movement.

**4.** *Psychogenic.* When this is suspected the benefit of the doubt must be given to the patient. Psychogenic back pain is rare and only when every other source has been ruled out must this be given serious consideration.

*Note:* Metastasis from a primary source of cancer can cause unremitting back pain. If a patient complains of pain that is not relieved by rest it is conceivable that part of the past history has been missed.

## SUMMARY

This chapter began with Idiopathic Scoliosis which is a common affliction of the thoracic spine. Osteoporosis, which occurs in various parts of the skeletal framework, was included in this chapter because of its frequency in the thoracic spine. The section on the thoracic spine terminated with a discussion of disc disorders.

At the beginning of the section on the lumbar spine the reader was referred back to Chapter 2 for anatomy relating to the functional unit, the intervertebral foramen,and other pertinent anatomical aspects; although there are distinct differences there are some similarities between the anatomy of the cervical spine and the lumbar spine. However, it was thought necessary to spend some time on the lumbar zygapophyseal joints, the variation that exists in the orientation of their articular surfaces,and the effect of this variation on movement control.

The conditions discussed included common Lumbar Disc Lesions and the full root syndromes, Lumbar Spondylosis, Stenosis (including a comparison of symptomatology between it and disc lesions) Spondylolisis and Spondylolisthesis, Zygapophyseal Joint Problems, and Lumbosacral Strain. The chapter concluded with a discussion of some Sacroiliac Problems and Non-Musculoskeletal Causes of Low Back Pain.

# CHAPTER 6

# An Introduction to the McKenzie Approach to the Examination and Treatment of Low Back Pain

McKenzie (1981) is a proponent of the "hands off" approach to the treatment of low back pain (LBP) unless the patient's problem warrants the intervention of manual therapy or other treatment approaches. He has identified the main causes of LBP as postural problems (the **Postural Syndrome**), shortening of soft tissue structures (the **Dysfunction Syndrome**), and disc pathology (the **Derangement Syndrome**).

The predisposing factors, which are responsible for the onset of these syndromes, relate largely to the flexed position, the frequency of the adoption of the flexed position, and the resulting loss of extension. In addition, there are certain precipitating factors that include unexpected movements and incorrect lifting techniques.

## THE SYNDROMES

This chapter introduces each of the three syndromes in terms of cause, underlying pathology, and distinctive clinical features; treatment guidelines complete each section.

## THE POSTURAL SYNDROME

The postural syndrome results from stretching of soft tissues (mechanical deformation) caused by prolonged postural stresses. It is characterized by pain that occurs **only** on the maintenance of a given poor posture. The pain ceases when the stretching of the soft tissues is terminated by changing position. For instance, if slouch sitting is maintained during an evening of watching television, pain will result because of stretching of the posterior spinal soft tissue structures. This pain is relieved by sitting upright, with retention of the normal lordosis, thus taking the stretch off the posterior structures.

## Treatment Guidelines

Treatment quidelines consist of:

- educating the patient regarding the cause of the LBP and of generally poor postural habits, and
- teaching the patient how to achieve and retain a good posture, particularly in the sitting position.

### Educating the Patient

Patients are often aware that their LBP occurs only after sitting in a slouched position for a given length of time; however, they are unaware of the prolonged stress on the posterior structures that is giving rise to their pain; it is important to educate them in this regard. It is equally important to emphasize the significance of maintaining a normal lordosis at all times, and to identify for the patient poor postural habits in standing and lying and how to correct them.

### Teaching the Patient How to Achieve and Maintain a Good Posture

The process begins by the therapist explaining the points regarding good postural positions.

The patient is allowed to assume the slouched position until the LBP appears. The therapist then causes an over-correction by standing in front of the patient and placing his or her hands on the patient's lumbar spine and passively moving it into extension beyond the normal lordosis. The patient is encouraged in awareness of this position that may cause a new discomfort. Next, he or she is eased out of **this** over-corrected position until a normal lordosis is achieved and awareness of **this** position is internalized. The process is repeated. Retention of the lordotic position is facilitated by the utilization of a lumbar roll.

# THE DYSFUNCTION SYNDROME

Adaptive shortening of soft tissue structures, with ensuing loss of movement, develops as a result of habitual poor posture, disc lesions, or trauma. Pain is created when the shortened structures are stretched at the end of the available range of motion. The syndrome is described in terms of the movement that is restricted. If extension of the back causes pain at the end of the available range of motion the patient would be exhibiting an **extension dysfunction**. Similarly, if flexion causes pain at the end of the available range, a **flexion dysfunction** would be present. A chronic postural syndrome can develop into a dysfunction syndrome if the former is ignored.

## Treatment Guidelines

Much of what was presented under the treatment of postural problems should be applied if the problem is an extension dysfunction. However, the patient could have a flexion dysfunction and this will involve

- teaching the patient exercises that will enable the adaptive shortening of the dorsal soft tissue structures to be gently stretched without causing microtrauma.

The exercises should, however, cause some discomfort across the low back; otherwise no stretching is taking place.

### Teaching the Exercises

Restoration of function from a flexion dysfunction will not occur overnight and the patient must be told that the longer the problem has been in existence the longer it will take to restore range of motion. The patient is instructed in flexion in lying (Figure 6–1: position 3) to be performed ten times approximately every two hours. When full movement has been achieved with this exercise, in about 6 days, flexion in standing is used to regain maximum functional lumbar flexion. It is suggested that because flexion in standing is a vulnerable position (particularly if the dysfunction is associated with a derangement syndrome) the patient should perform only about six exercises five or six times a day.

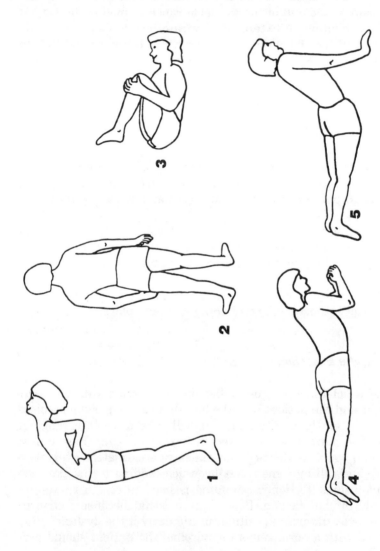

**Figure 6–1.** (1) Extension in standing; (2) Left side glide; (3) Flexion in supine; (4) Lying prone in extension; and (5) Extension in prone lying (adapted from McKenzie, 1981).

## THE DERANGEMENT SYNDROME

In the previous chapter disc protrusions with full nerve root involvement were described. McKenzie (1981) hypothesizes about what happens within the disc prior to the development of the protrusion and beyond and describes the process as a derangement.

A derangement is abnormal movement between the articular surfaces of the intervertebral joint because of changes in the position of the nucleus. Repetitive or prolonged flexion stresses, accompanied by an increase in intradiscal pressure, force the nucleus in a posterior direction thus exerting stress on the inner walls of the annulus. The collagen fibers of the annulus give way and the nuclear material seeps through, interfering with the normal movement between the articular surfaces and causing a painful derangement. If the process of seepage continues, a protrusion of the outer wall of the annulus is formed with possible pressure on the nerve root as described in the previous chapter. Once again a derangement syndrome and a dysfunction syndrome may co-exist because of repair of damage following a derangement.

McKenzie discusses different derangements and their clinical features that will be described later and related to the disc lesion symptomatology described in the previous chapter.

## THE EXAMINATION

In order to determine the cause of the patient's LBP, subjective and objective examinations are performed. Questions relating to the former will be discussed next.

### The Subjective Examination

During the subjective examination the patient is asked meaningful and concise questions; the therapist should **listen attentively to the responses** (Edwardson, 1992).

*How old are you?* The postural syndrome develops **before** the age of 30 years, the dysfunction syndrome usually develops **after** the age of 30, and the derangement syndrome develops **between** the ages of 20 and 55.

*What is your position at work?* A slouched sitting position could indicate a postural syndrome or a dysfunction syndrome; referred pain on sitting could be indicative of a derangement.

*Where is the present pain felt? Is the pain associated with anesthesia, paresthesia, or numbness?* Referred symptoms and neurological signs are indicative of a derangement.

*Has the pain always been where you feel it now?* Pain that moves from one side of the back to the other or moves into the leg is indicative of a derangement.

*How long has the pain been present?* (Is the condition acute, subacute, or chronic?) The condition may be recurrent. If so, the present episode becomes the focus of examination. The longer the problem has been in existence the greater are the chances of dysfunction being present. The length of time the pain has been present gives some indication of how vigorous the objective examination can be. If it has been present for a short time and is constant, great care is taken in handling the patient. If the condition has been in existence for months, a more vigorous approach can be used.

*How did the pain start? What caused it?* If the patient does not know how the pain started it is possible that a derangement or dysfunction has developed during the course of normal daily living. Severe pain that occurs in the flexed position and prevents the patient from straightening up is indicative of a derangement. If, however, the pain started for **no apparent reason**, is constant and **getting worse**, serious pathology must be suspected, particularly if the patient does not feel or look well.

*Is the pain intermittent or constant?* Intermittent pain is always produced by mechanical deformation. If it is constant it is caused by constant mechanical deformation or chemical irritation. Intermittent pain is easier to treat. The derangement syndrome is likely to produce constant pain whereas the postural and dysfunction syndromes are likely to produce intermittent pain.

*What makes the pain worse, what makes the pain better?* If **standing** in the relaxed position makes the pain worse, it is evident that sustained extension is causing mechanical deformation. If the patient finds relief in relaxed standing, then extension reduces the mechanical deformation. Similarly, if the patient complains of pain in relaxed **sitting** then flexion is causing mechanical deformation; if the patient is comfortable in relaxed sitting, flexion eases the mechanical deformation. **Walking** causes an increase in the lordosis and if the patient's pain is eased by walking then extension is decreasing the mechanical deformation. The reverse is the case if walking increases the patient's pain. Finally, the **lying** position can provide information regarding its influence on pain. The patient may be either in prone, where the spine is near maximum extension, supine where the spine can either fall into extension (firm mattress), or flexion (soft mattress), or side lying where the lumbar spine goes into a lateral curvature with the convexity on the side on which the patient is lying.

*Have there been previous episodes of low back pain?* Previous episodes of constant LBP indicate a derangement.

The mandatory questions regarding medication, general health, recent weight loss, saddle anesthesia, and similar factors are also asked.

## The Objective Examination

The objective examination commences with observation of the patient in different positions, where note is taken of any deviation from the norm, and continues with testing of the patient's movements.

### Observation

It is important to observe the patient's posture in sitting and standing.

*Sitting:*                      Is there a **slouch**?

*Standing:*              Is there a **reduced or accentuated lordosis**?

Is there a **lateral shift** of the spine to the right or left causing a scoliosis? A left lateral shift is present if the left shoulder and the trunk are positioned beyond the left hip and pelvis (Figure 6–1: position 2). Note: In a diagram a left lateral shift and a left side glide would appear the same.

Is there **leg length discrepancy** (LLD)? LLD is not significant if there is no pain in standing or walking.

### Examination of Movement

Initially the integrity of the L5 nerve root is tested by asking tne patient to lean back on the heels and the integrity of nerve root S1 is tested by asking the patient to stand on the toes. Weakness in performance with successive tests indicates interference in nerve root conductivity and the presence of a derangement.

## Single Test Movements

The following three movements are performed once only in standing and the examiner takes note of the quality of each movement.

**1.** *Flexion.* This test provides the examiner with the most relevant information regarding the nature and extent of the derangement or dysfunction. The patient is asked to bend forward as far as possible, running the fingertips down the front of the legs, then returning **immediately** to the neutral standing position. Loss of flexion manifests itself in two ways, as described below.

(i) The end of range is limited; instead of the normal rounding of the lumbar spine that should occur on forward flexion, the examiner will see a lordotic or flat lumbar spine.

(ii) There may be deviation from the normal sagittal pathway of forward flexion to one side, indicating one of the following conditions:

- a derangement within the joint with the deviation usually **away from** the painful side;
- dysfunction in the joint because of adaptive shortening following repair of damage after a derangement; this causes a deviation **toward** the side of the dysfunction;
- dysfunction external to the joint because of a tethered nerve root; this will cause deviation in the direction that will not stretch the tethered nerve root.

**2.** *Extension.* The patient is asked to place the backs of the hands in the lumbar region and extend backwards as far as possible (Figure 6–1: position 1). Some loss of extension is normal after the age of 40 years; however, its presence should be recorded. The loss of movement could be attributable to a posterior buildup of the fluid nucleus, to an extension dysfunction, or to the presence of a lateral shift.

**3.** *Side Gliding.* This is a combination of rotation and side flexion. The patient is asked to move the shoulders and pelvis simultaneously in opposite directions in a horizontal plane. In the presence of a lateral shift there is always some loss of movement to the side **opposite** to that of the lateral shift.

## Repeated Test Movements

Following the single performance of the above three exercises the patient is instructed in repeated test movements.

The following five movements are performed repeatedly. Except for the first movement which is self-explanatory the movements are illustrated in Figure 6–1. Extension in prone (Figure 6–1: position 4) is also shown as this is often an intermediate stage of repeated extension in lying (Figure 6–1: position 5).

1. *Repeated Forward Flexion in Standing*
2. *Repeated Extension in Standing*
3. *Repeated Side Gliding in Standing*
4. *Repeated Flexion in Lying*—The patient brings the knees to the chest; "pressure on," then "pressure off."
5. *Repeated Extension in Lying*—The patient performs a push-up with the elbows fully extending; "up," then "down."

When performing the above movements it is important that the patient goes as far as possible with each movement then returns quickly to the starting position. Instructions are specific: for example, "Bend forwards as far as you can, now come up." The therapist ensures that the patient's feet are more than hip width apart for all movements in standing. After the first careful performance of the exercise the therapist asks "What has happened to your pain?" If pain is not increased, the patient does three or four more repetitions; the therapist then asks "What has happened now?"

The test movement may be repeated approximately ten times, providing the symptoms are not becoming increasingly worse.

### Movements in Relation to Pain

*Test Movements in Standing.* **A normal stress is applied** to normal or abnormal tissue.

*Test Movements in Lying.* **A passive stress is added** by the patient, thus, an **abnormal stress is applied** to normal or abnormal tissue. In the normal tissue no pain should develop because the movement is momentary. In the abnormal tissue mechanical deformation is enhanced, and pain is produced. However, pain will be decreased or abolished if the movement reduces the mechanical deformation.

If movements are to be related to pain, **the test movements must be performed in such a way as to produce a change in the patient's symptoms. If pain is present** before the test, the test may increase or decrease it; it may alter its site; or the pain could be abolished and another produced. **If no pain is present** the movement may produce the pain complained of. If the movements do not change the patient's symptoms, the therapist should consider the following possibilities:

- the exercises have not been performed vigorously enough and should be repeated; or
- the pain is not of mechanical origin; or
- the lumbar spine is not causing the problems and some other cause should be sought.

### The Significance of the Repeated Movements

The movements are particularly important when **disc pathology** is suspected. McKenzie (1981) believes that movement of the vertebral column causes an alteration in the shape of the nucleus and that repeated movements and/or sustained movement eventually alter the position of the nucleus.

A disc protrusion of sufficient size will cause pressure on the nerve root and dura mater, creating pain and paresthesia extending below the knee. As the protrusion reduces in size as a result of selected movements, the pressure on these sensitive structures is released, the pain and paresthesia below the knee disappear, and there is a reduction in thigh pain. The focus of the pain is now in the buttock or lumbar region. This reversal of symptoms is called the **centralization phenomenon** and the movements which brought it about are those that will be used in treatment.

Conversely, movements can increase the size of the protrusion, and pain, initially felt in the lumbar region, extends down the back of the leg with accompanying paresthesia. When this occurs, the protrusion has increased in size and the resulting phenomenon is called **peripheralization**. The movements that caused it to happen, for instance repeated flexion, are avoided in treatment, and movements in the opposite direction (extension) are selected instead.

Repeated movements are also useful in the **diagnosis of a dysfunction** when used in the direction which stretches the shortened structures. Pain is produced at the end of range for each movement, but repeated movements do not make the patient worse.

Patients with a **postural syndrome** will not have pain with any of the test movements.

When repeated movements applied to painful structures produce less and less pain these movements should be used. If more and more pain is produced with repeated movements more healing time should be allowed.

### Flexion in Standing Versus Flexion in Lying

In flexion in lying (Figure 6–1: position 3) there is no gravitational stress and flexion begins at L5-S1 then ascends the spine. In flexion in standing, movement begins at L1 and descends to L4. A better flexion stretch is obtained at the L5-S1 level in passive flexion in lying. Stretching of L4-5-S1 during flexion in standing only occurs when the flexion is almost complete.

The sciatic nerve is fully stretched in flexion in standing. Enhancement of sciatic pain in this position may be caused by a bulging disc or an adherent root. Enhancement of sciatic pain in lying can only be caused by a bulging disc. **WE NOW HAVE A SIMPLE TEST TO DIFFERENTIATE BETWEEN DISC BULGING AND ADHERENT ROOT.**

### Extension in Standing Versus Extension in Lying

In extension in lying, the weight of the pelvis and abdomen causes an increase in extension range and the greatest extension stretch is achieved.

In extension in standing, the compression forces appear to be sufficient to prevent full end-range movement. This indicates that some derangements are too large to be reduced in the presence of compressive forces. Reduction of these derangements becomes possible when the compressive forces are reduced by extension in lying.

*Note:* If no position or movement during the examination can be found which reduces the presenting pain the patient is considered unsuitable for mechanical therapy. Such a patient is usually in the acute stage and in a great deal of pain caused by compressive forces in the standing or sitting position. Bed rest is recommended prior to treatment. Even so, reassessment should be performed after 48 hours to determine whether the patient would then respond to treatment by movement or positioning.

Further detail regarding specific derangements will be discussed next.

## TABLE OF DERANGEMENTS

McKenzie (1981) has classified the derangements into seven types. The first six derangements are increasingly severe stages of the first posterior derangement and should be treated utilizing the extension principle; the seventh is an anterior derangement, treated by the flexion principle.

## DERANGEMENT 1

Derangement 1 is a minor displacement of disc material in a posterocentral direction.

### Clinical Features

- Central or symmetrical pain across L4/5
- Rarely buttock or thigh pain
- No deformity

## DERANGEMENT 2

In Derangement 2 a deformity is present caused by posterocentral accumulation of nuclear material and care must be taken with treatment to avoid an acute lateral shift.

### Clinical Features

- As above with or without buttock and/or thigh pain
- Presence of a lumbar kyphosis

## DERANGEMENT 3

In Derangement 3 the changes within the disc are in a posterolateral direction rather than a posterocentral direction.

### Clinical Features

- Unilateral or asymmetrical pain across L4/L5
- Buttock and/or thigh pain may or may not be present
- No deformity

## DERANGEMENT 4

McKenzie regards Derangement 4 as a lateral progression of Derangement 2 and a simple progression of Derangement 3.

### Clinical Features

The clinical features for this derangement are as above but a deformity is present in the form of **a lumbar scoliosis** (lateral shift).

## DERANGEMENT 5

Derangement 5 is a progression of Derangement 3.

### Clinical Features

The clinical features for this derangement are the same as for Derangement 3 **but leg pain, which extends below the knee, is present.** There is no deformity.

## DERANGEMENT 6

Derangement 6 is a progression of Derangements 4 and 5.

### Clinical Features

The clinical features are the same as for Derangement 4 **but leg pain is present and extends below the knee**. A sciatic scoliosis is present.

## DERANGEMENT 7

Derangement 7 is uncommon and the disc material appears to travel in an anterior or anterolateral direction, limiting forward flexion. A lumbar lordosis is evident on completion of the available range of forward flexion.

## Clinical Features

- Asymmetrical or symmetrical pain across L4/L5
- Buttock and/or thigh pain that may or may not be present
- Presence of an accentuated lumbar lordosis

## Treatment Guidelines

The philosophy of treatment involves three principles:

1. reduction of the derangement;
2. maintenance of the reduction;
3. recovery of full function.

In terms of relating McKenzie's test movements to the treatment of patients, only the displacements in a posterior direction, which respond to a hands-off approach, will be discussed.

### 1. Reduction of the Derangement

It was stated earlier that the repeated test movements that relieve the patient's pain will be selected for treatment purposes. With minor derangements in a posterior direction the first exercise of **lying prone** for at least five minutes is followed by the second exercise of **lying prone in extension in the forearm support position** (Figure 6–1: position 4); these positions are used to facilitate reduction of the disc material. In the latter position the patient allows the lumbar spine to "sag," achieving an increased lordosis, for a similar period of time.

In more severe displacements, where a kyphosis is present, the patient may be unable to lie in the prone position initially and may have to lie prone over pillows in order to achieve some reduction of the disc material. When the patient is able to lie comfortably in the prone position over pillows the pillows are gradually removed and he or she is allowed to progress to lying prone in extension as indicated above.

If the patient is unable to tolerate sustained extension in prone lying with forearm support for at least five minutes he or she is encouraged to move intermittently from lying prone to lying prone in extension with forearm support. The third repeated exercise is **extension in lying** (Figure 6–1: position 5) which is a "pushup" to the elbow-extended position with care being taken to ensure that the pelvis remains in contact with the treatment table. The patient is encouraged to perform the exercises up to ten times every waking hour for 24 hours. The repeated exercises can be reduced to three times a day as the reduction is maintained and can be discontinued when the constant pain has subsided.

In minor displacements of the disc material, lying prone in extension may be sufficient to produce a reduction and there is no need to progress to fuller extension in lying.

### 2. Maintenance of the Reduction

Instruction in postural correction in terms of maintaining the normal lordosis **at all times** is essential in this part of the treatment program. However, the correction does not commence from the slouched position, as in the postural syndrome, since in this position the spine is in flexion. Instruction and demonstration in moving from the lying position, or sitting position, to the standing position without allowing the spine to lose the lordosis are an important part of the program. The use of the lumbar roll will facilitate the maintenance of the normal lordosis in the sitting position.

### 3. Recovery of Full Function

Because of the frequency of posterior derangements and their treatment with extension exercises it is sometimes erroneously assumed that McKenzie is "the extension guru." In this stage of the treatment program flexion in lying is gradually introduced; when the patient is able to reach maximum range of flexion in lying he or she can progress to flexion in standing. Full recovery has occurred when the patient can achieve full range of flexion in the standing position without pain.

### Manual Techniques in Extension and Rotation

Sometimes a patient will make progress with repeated extension movements in the treatment of a posterior derangement and will then appear to plateau. In such cases manual therapy in terms of mobilization in extension or rotation may bring about the desired result. Manual extension may be applied before the plateau is reached to hasten recovery. However, where possible, laying on of hands should be avoided so that the patient is independent of the therapist and in charge of his own treatment.

Cyriax (1982) has found that forced extension is suitable for L4 disc lesions and that a rotation manipulation is beneficial for L5 disc lesions; he believed in the early manipulative approach to treatment rather than the "treat yourself approach" advocated by McKenzie.

### Corrective Procedure for the Patient with Deviation to the Right on Forward Flexion

If a patient is seen to deviate to the **right** in forward flexion because of either a dysfunction, a tethered nerve root, or a derangement, the **left** foot should be placed on a chair so that the hip and knee are at 90°; the right leg remains straight and on the ground. The patient bends forward so that the left knee and left shoulder are approximating and the hands are gripping around the leg towards the ankle. Further range may be obtained by flexing the elbow and gripping around the ankle, allowing the head and left shoulder to flex even more. The procedure should be repeated several times BUT after each exercise the spine should be allowed to go into extension.

*Rationale for the Above:* Asymmetrically shortened structures are stretched in the dysfunction. In the derangement, the nucleus is moved to a central position from a position in the lateral compartment.

## SUMMARY

This chapter began with a definition of the three syndromes, predisposing factors, and participating factors as described by McKenzie (1981). This was followed by a more detailed description of the three syndromes in terms of their underlying pathology, clinical features, and treatment guidelines. Next, the subjective and objective examinations were discussed and the findings were interpreted for the reader. Finally, the different derangements were identified in terms of their clinical features, and the treatment approaches were discussed in terms of reducing the derangement, maintaining the reduction, and restoring full function.

CHAPTER 7

• • • • • • • •

# The Hip Region

The hip joint is one of the most stable joints in the body. Unlike its counterpart, the glenohumeral joint in the upper extremity whose prime function is mobility, the articular surfaces of the hip joint achieve almost complete congruence. Steindler (1955) has shown that complete congruence of the hip is achieved in the positions of flexion, abduction, and external rotation. In the upright position the anterior portion of the head of the femur is not covered by the acetabulum. Soderberg (1986) identifies the deficiency as being on the anterosuperior surface of the femoral head. The hip is also well supported by ligaments; additional bony architectural aspects of the hip joint contribute to the stability, namely, the **angle of inclination** and the **angle of anteversion**. The contribution of all these stabilizing factors is necessary for the hip to perform its weightbearing function.

The hip is closely associated with the pelvis, and some biomechanical aspects relating to the pelvis, as well as repetitive strain disorders relating to this structure, will also be included in this chapter.

## BIOMECHANICS IN SINGLE LEG STANCE

In single leg stance, the center of the weightbearing hip joint acts as a fulcrum (F) between two unequal lever arms in a first class lever system (Figure 7–1). The longest lever arm (a) is the distance from (F) to the vertical line of the body weight (BW). The shorter lever arm (b) is the distance from (F) to the vertical line of the force

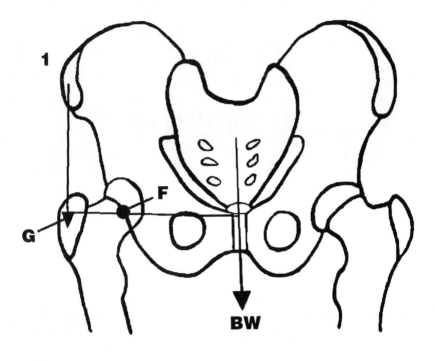

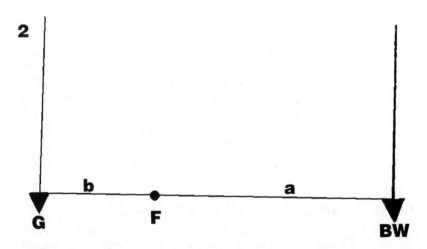

**Figure 7–1.** Moments of force about the stance hip: (1) Anatomical representation; (2) biomechanical model; (F) center of the hip joint (the fulcrum); (G) gluteal force; (BW) location and direction of body weight; (a) gluteal lever arm; (b) body weight lever arm (adapted from Le Veau, 1977).

(G) exerted by the abductor muscles, gluteus medius and minimus. This muscle group works from its stable insertion on the greater trochanter of the femur to pull downwards on its origin from the pelvic rim in order to prevent the pelvis on the side of the non-weightbearing leg from dropping.

The moment of force exerted about an axis is the product of the lever arm and the applied force or weight. A consideration of the diagram representing the two uneven lever arms (Figure 7–1), as viewed from the front, indicates that an anticlockwise moment (negative) is created by the abductor muscles and a clockwise moment (positive) is created by the body weight. In order for the body to achieve equilibrium the sum of the moments of the two lever systems must equal zero, that is :

$$BW \times a + (-G \times b) = 0$$

OR

$$BW \times a = G \times b$$

If we assume that the distance (a) is twice that of distance (b), and that BW = 80 kgm, then the abductor force (G) can be calculated as follows:

$$80 \times 2 = G \times 1$$
$$160 = G$$

The total load on the center of the hip joint would be:

$$80 + 160 = 240 \text{ kgm.}$$

The above concept has important implications, as will be seen later, when we consider ways in which a patient will try to decrease the pain, for example in an osteoarthritic hip. The patient will attempt to equalize the length of the two lever arms thus reducing the total load on the hip.

## SIGNIFICANT ANGLES

During embryonic development, and following birth, the shaft of the femur assumes a position of inward rotation and adduction which causes the head and neck of the femur to form angles with the shaft of the femur in the frontal and horizontal planes. The angle the head and neck form in the frontal plane is called the **angle of inclination** (Figure 7–2: diagram 1) and the angle formed by the head and neck in the horizontal plane is the **angle of anteversion** (Figure 7–2: diagram 2).

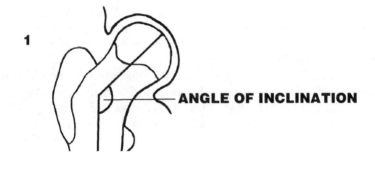

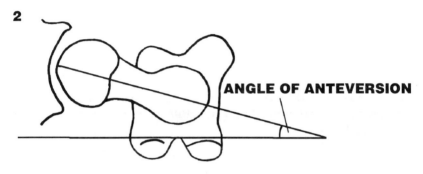

**Figure 7–2.** Significant angles of the hip joint: (1) angle of inclination; (2) angle of anteversion (adapted from Oatis, 1990).

## The Angle of Inclination

The **angle of inclination** represents the adaptation the femur has made in going from the abducted position in the embryo, to the adducted position in upright stance in order to ensure that the legs are parallel (Steindler,1955). In the newborn the angle measures 150° but this decreases to an angle of 125° in the adult (Figure 7–3: diagram 1).

An increase in the angle of inclination is called **coxa valga** (Figure 7–3: diagram 2) and if present unilaterally it will produce an increase in limb length on the affected side with accompanying **genu varum**. The body compensates for this increase at the pelvis, the ankle, and the foot. Because the anatomical and mechanical axes are closer together in coxa valga there is **less stress on the femoral neck**. There is, however, an **increased load on the hip joint**, because of the decrease in length of the abductor lever arm.

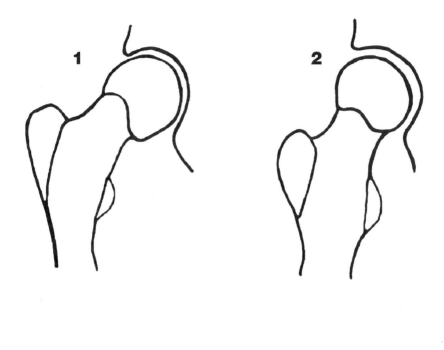

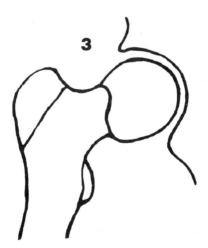

**Figure 7–3.** Normal and abnormal angles of inclination: (1) normal position; (2) coxa valga—increased angle of inclination; (3) coxa vara—decreased angle of inclination.

Conversely, a decrease in the angle of inclination is called **coxa vara** (Figure 7–3: diagram 3), resulting in a decrease in limb length on the affected side with accompanying **genu valgum**, for which the body will again compensate to some extent. Because the anatomical and mechanical axes are further apart in coxa vara there will be **greater stress on the femoral neck**. Because the abductor lever arm is increased in length, as a result of a decrease in the angle of inclination, there will be **less load on the hip joint** (Oatis, 1990).

## The Angle of Anteversion

In the horizontal plane there is an angle between the neck and the shaft of the femur called the **angle of anteversion** (Figure 7–2: diagram 2). This angle was created by the head and neck rotating laterally against the shaft and the shaft remaining in medial rotation against the neck of the femur (Steindler, 1955). The angle can be observed if the femoral bone is placed on a table so that the condyles of the femur are in contact with the table. If the femur is observed from the head end, at eye level to the table, it will be noted that the head and neck of the femur rotate outwards on the shaft creating the angle of anteversion. The angle represents the change in the shaft of the femur from outward rotation to inward rotation in the normal standing position. The average angle of anteversion, from an extensive study performed by Kingsley in 1948 and cited by Steindler (1955), was found to be 8.021 degrees in the adult. An excessively large angle may be a factor in the "miserable malalignment syndrome" discussed in the next chapter.

## MOVEMENTS OF THE PELVIS

The movements of the pelvis are discussed below.

- Anterior and posterior rotations in a transverse plane occur when one half of the pelvis is either ahead of, or behind, the other half of the pelvis. Anterior rotation accompanies flexion in gait and posterior rotation accompanies extension.
- Anterior and posterior tilts occur in a saggital plane. The anterior superior iliac spines (ASIS) move bilaterally in a forward and downward direction with an anterior tilt and upwards and backwards in a posterior tilt.
- Lateral tilts of the pelvis are described as elevation or depression. Elevation is accompanied by trunk side flexion to

the same side and adduction of the elevated hip. Depression is accompanied by trunk side flexion to the opposite side and by hip abduction.

## CONDITIONS IN THE HIP REGION

There are a number of abnormal conditions that develop in and around the hip joint. Many of these are soft tissue in nature, but the most prevalent is a degenerative condition of the joint called osteoarthritis, which will be discussed next.

## OSTEOARTHRITIS

Osteoarthritis is the most common affliction of the hip joint in persons over the age of 50 years. In spite of this the cause remains obscure and there does not appear to be a good correlation between the amount of pain experienced by the patient and the extent of the pathological changes (Threlkeld & Currier, 1988). The condition varies tremendously in degree and progression (Turek, 1984).

### Etiology

At least 50 per cent of the cases of osteoarthritis are idiopathic in nature, but the degenerative changes could be accelerated by certain imposed conditions (Turek, 1984). Some of these imposed conditions are listed below.

- Coxa vara or excessive anteversion, either of which could lead to a concentration of pressure on part of the head of the femur
- Incongruity of articular surfaces caused by, for instance, subluxation
- Trauma
- Obesity
- Congenital disorders, such as congenital dislocation of the hip or Perthe's disease

### Pathology

The pathology of this condition is not fully understood. Degeneration of the articular cartilage is known to occur, but this can be present without any clinical manifestation such as pain (Threlkeld & Currier, 1988). The degenerative pathology of the cartilage and sub-chondral bone is as follows:

- degeneration of the articular cartilage;
- inflammation, following the establishment of degenerative changes;
- sclerosis of the subchondral bone with eburnation;
- osteophyte formation;
- loss of joint space;
- cyst formation.

Threlkeld and Currier (1988) have drawn attention to the soft tissue involvement in osteoarthritis:

- thickening and increased vascularity of the synovial membrane;
- thickening of the joint capsule and distention;
- fraying of ligamentum teres;
- muscle atrophy;
- impairment of joint position sense;
- inconsistent stimulation of the nociceptor system in surrounding tissues.

## Clinical Features

Pain is the clinical feature that will cause the patient to seek med-ical or surgical help. It manifests itself, albeit inconsistently, in one of the following areas, or in a combination of areas:

- over the greater trochanter and/or the medial gluteal region;
- the groin, anterior thigh, the knee, and down the tibia.

Other clinical features are:

- joint effusion and muscle spasm;
- an antalgic gait; the patient attempts to decrease the load on the hip (and thus decrease the pain) by lurching towards the affected side on weightbearing (refer to the biomechanics);
- muscle atrophy, particularly of the abductor muscles;
- loss of joint range in extension, abduction, and internal rotation;
- development of a flexion, adduction, and external rotation deformity.

## Treatment Guidelines

Treatment involves a multifaceted approach and is aimed at decreasing the pain and maintaining range of motion and muscle strength. Various techniques have been described to achieve these ends and they will not be repeated here (Grieve, 1983; Kaltenborn, 1989; Lee, 1989; Maitland, 1991).

The use of assistive devices, such as a cane held in the hand on the contralateral side, will decrease the load on the hip joint. Carrying a weight, such as a suitcase, in the hand on the same side as the affected hip will achieve similar results (Neumann & Cook, 1985). Equalization of limb length utilizing a lift in the shoe on the short side will help decrease the excessive joint forces and consequently the pain (Echternach, 1990).

There must be a balance between weightbearing activities and rest and the patient must be educated in this regard.

## Surgical Intervention

Total hip replacement is one of the most common and successful surgical procedures carried out today. Following surgery the patient remains in hospital for a few days during which time he or she is taught exercises by a physical therapist to perform during the hospital stay. The exercises are progressed under supervision when the patient leaves hospital. The aims of such a program are to rid the patient of old habit patterns, and to develop strength and flexibility in the new range.

## BURSITIS

There are a large number of bursae associated with the hip region; the function of these is to reduce friction between adjacent soft tissue structures such as tendon and muscle or between tendon and bone. The bursae are small sacs that have a lining similar to synovium and are vulnerable to any inflammatory condition affecting synovial joints such as rheumatoid arthritis (Lotke, 1991).

The most common cause of bursitis, unassociated with inflammatory conditions of the hip joint, relates to their function as friction reducers. Repetitive stress on the bursa from a tight overlying structure can produce an inflammatory response. Two common problems associated with bursae are discussed below.

## A. TROCHANTERIC BURSITIS

The bursae which are most frequently involved in this way are the superficial and deep trochanteric bursae (Figure 7–4). The superficial trochanteric bursa lies beneath the fascia lata on the upper lateral part of the greater trochanter; the deep trochanteric bursa lies between the gluteus medius tendon and the posterior part of the greater trochanter (Peterson & Renstrom, 1986).

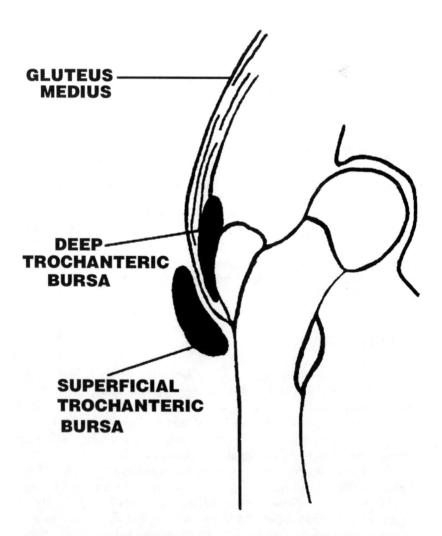

**GLUTEUS MEDIUS**

**DEEP TROCHANTERIC BURSA**

**SUPERFICIAL TROCHANTERIC BURSA**

**Figure 7–4.** Trochanteric bursae.

## Mechanism of Injury

Joggers who run on the camber of the road or who have pronated feet can subject either bursa to repetitive stress resulting in an inflammatory response.

## Clinical Features

The clinical features are as follows:

- tenderness on palpation over the upper lateral part of the thigh;
- pain that is experienced over the upper lateral aspect of the thigh and may extend down the thigh;
- an increase in pain on resisted abduction or passive adduction.

## Treatment Guidelines

If the condition is caught in its early stages it may respond to rest, ice, and correction of an adverse running style. An orthotic device would be helpful in correcting pronation if this is a predisposing cause.

Medical treatment involves aspiration, and injections of analgesics and steroids. Surgical excision may be necessary.

*Note:* Other bursae which less frequently become inflamed, are the **iliopsoas bursa**, the **ischial bursa**, and the **iliopectineal bursa**. Symptoms will be related to the location of the bursa.

## B. SNAPPING HIP

Snapping hip problem is closely associated with the trochanteric bursa. It is characterized by a snapping sound on certain movements of the hip, which may, or may not, be accompanied by pain. When it is accompanied by pain it implicates an associated bursa and warrants investigation.

## Etiology

The causes can be intra-articular or extra-articular. The condition arises more frequently from extra-articular than from intra-articular causes; the latter are not clearly understood. The most common extra-articular causes among the former are the iliotibial band or tract (Figure 7–5) slipping over the greater trochanter and the anter-

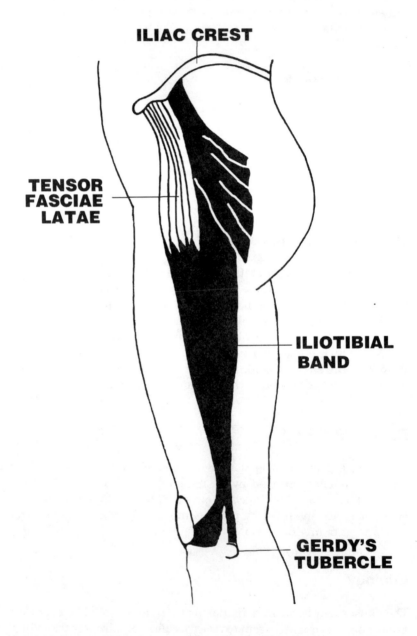

**Figure 7–5.** Iliotibial band and its attachments.

ior border of the gluteus maximus slipping over the greater trochanter (Schaberg, Harper, & Allen, 1984). The iliopsoas tendon slipping over the iliopectineal eminence has been cited as another common extra-articular cause. Intra-articular causes include loose bodies in the joint and subluxation of the hip (Zoltan, Clancy, & Keene, 1986).

## Clinical Features

The painful symptoms invariably relate to an inflammation of the associated bursa as a result of repetitive stresses. The condition is most common in adolescents and young women and is often associated with a nervous habit of rotating the leg; the patient can reproduce the snapping sound by flexing and internally rotating the thigh (Lotke,1991).

- There is an audible snapping sound.
- There will be pain and tenderness over the site of the trochanteric bursa and the pain may be referred down the thigh.
- Movements associated with compression of the bursa will increase the pain.

## Treatment Guidelines

If the condition is asymptomatic no treatment is warranted other than advising avoidance of movements that will produce the snapping sound. Stretchings of a tight structure, such as the iliotibial band, are helpful. If the bursa is involved the condition is treated as a bursitis (see trochanteric bursitis above). Surgical intervention, for instance release of the iliotibial band, may be necessary in chronic cases.

## TENDINITIS AND MUSCLE RUPTURES

The increase in physical activity over the past few years has brought with it joys and sorrows. High on the list of the latter is the increase in soft tissue injuries and those associated with the hip joint are no exception.

## A. TENDINITIS

Certain tendons, and/or their sheaths, around the hip joint are prone to injury with a resultant inflammatory response, as a result of overuse. The inflammatory response occurs at the insertion of the tendon. Palpation may not be easy, particularly if the traumatized tendon is deep. However, resisted isometric contractions of the suspected muscle should increase the pain and help to confirm the identity of the tendon at fault.

The **adductor longus tendon** often becomes inflamed at its origin on the pubic bone; the patient will present with local tenderness and increased pain on resisted adduction.

The **iliopsoas** can become inflamed at its insertion into the lesser trochanter. In this region it is associated with a bursa, which may also become inflamed. Resisted hip flexion will increase the pain associated with the condition.

The **rectus femoris** arises from two heads; the most proximal origin is from the anterior superior iliac spine and the distal origin arises from just above the acetabulum. It is the distal origin that can become inflamed through overuse. Resisted knee extension with the hip in neutral should increase the pain.

## B. MUSCLE RUPTURES

Muscle ruptures may occur in any of the muscles described above and the rupture may be partial or complete.

### Treatment Guidelines

Essentially the treatment approach for tendinitis and partial muscle rupture is that of rest, ice, compression, and anti-inflammatory medication followed by continuance of activities which do not cause pain. Progression of treatment involves a gradual return to training activities leading to full training activities.

For a complete rupture surgical repair may be implemented.

## OTHER PROBLEMS IN THE HIP AND PELVIC REGION ASSOCIATED WITH RUNNING

Brody (1980) has described other soft tissue injuries in the region of the hip and pelvis which can develop as a result of a faulty running style. Some of these are described briefly below.

## A. HAMSTRING STRAIN OR MUSCLE TEAR

Hamstring strain is a common problem associated with running and other forms of athletic activity. The injury can occur in the proximal tendinous part of the muscle, or in the middle or distal portion of the muscle. The injuries are treated with rest, ice, compression, and restoration of gentle movement when pain subsides.

## B. BUTTOCK PAIN

Pain in the buttock can develop as a result of a **tight piriformis muscle** compressing the sciatic nerve or from a **disc lesion** in the lower lumbar spine causing irritation of the associated nerve roots. In runners it is most likely caused by the latter. If it is attributable to tightness of the piriformis, stretching of the muscle is advocated.

## C. PELVIC DISORDERS

Painful disorders of the pelvis such as osteitis pubis, sacroiliitis, and iliac apophysitis develop as a result of repetitive stress caused by excessive pelvic motion. There can be **exaggeration of the anterior and posterior rotations** of the pelvis in the transverse plane if the runner's style involves the arms alternately moving **across** the chest. Uphill and downhill running can stress the pelvis because of excessive **tilting** of the pelvis in an **anterior and posterior direction**. Excessive mileage, or an inappropriate running style, can cause **excessive lateral tilting** of the pelvis.

In all the above conditions, correction of running style, in terms of appropriate increase in mileage, correction of the arm movement, appropriate footwear, and appropriate running terrain, is implemented following rest and anti-inflammatory medications.

## SUMMARY

Following a consideration of pertinent anatomy and biomechanics of the hip joint there was a discussion on the various aspects of Osteoarthritis of the hip joint. The latter is the most common malady of the hip joint affecting the middle aged and older person. Bursitis in the region of the hip joint was described followed by a discussion on the Snapping Hip syndrome. Tendinitis, muscle strains, and tears are common athletic injuries and examples of some of these were considered. The chapter concluded with consideration of problems affecting the pelvic joints since these are fairly common occurrences in joggers.

CHAPTER 8

• • • • • • • •

# The Patellofemoral Joint

Pain in and around the patellofemoral joint is a common finding, particularly in athletes. The joint is influenced by a number of soft tissue and bony factors (Brown, 1990; Rusche & Mangine, 1988; Welsh & Hutton, 1990a). A knowledge of these structures and their interaction with the patellofemoral joint is essential for correct diagnosis and treatment (Kramer, 1986; McConnell, 1986).

## BIOMECHANICAL FEATURES OF THE PATELLOFEMORAL JOINT

Normal tracking of the patella, a sinuous ascent from a medial position in flexion to a lateral position in extension (Helfet, 1974), is achieved by a delicate balance between medial and lateral soft tissue structures exerting a transverse pull and superior and inferior structures exerting a vertical pull (Figure 8–1). Under normal circumstances the pull of the lateral retinaculum, iliotibial band, and vastus lateralis is counteracted by the pull of the medial retinaculum and the oblique fibers of vastus medialis. In the vertical direction the main structures working together to achieve a balanced state are the quadriceps and the ligamentum patellae. Tightness of associated musculature such as rectus femoris, hamstrings, and gastrocnemius have also been reported to have an effect on the normal alignment of the patella (McConnell, 1986).

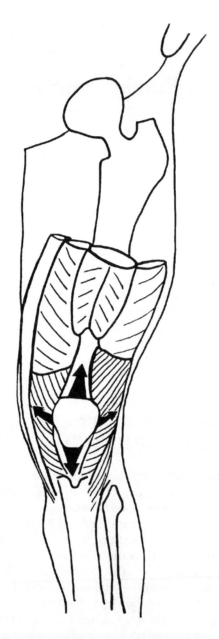

**Figure 8–1.** Stabilizing forces acting on the patella (adapted from Gill et al., 1991).

## The Q Angle

Apart from the soft tissue structures discussed above, other factors influence the normal tracking of the patella. The normal knee exhibits slight valgus (Nofthall, 1990; Welsh & Hutton, 1990a); this gives rise to the Q angle (Figure 8–2). This angle has a normal

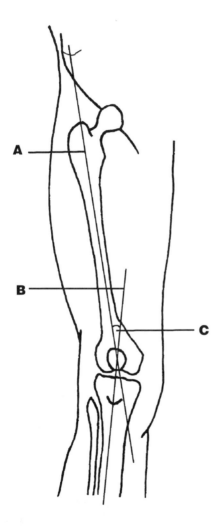

**Figure 8–2.**  The Q angle formed by intersecting lines: (A) a line from the ASIS through the center of the patella; (B) a line through the center of the patella and the long axis of the tibia; and (C) the Q angle.

range of 15–20° (Malek & Mangine, 1981), and exerts a lateral force on the patella; if this angle is abnormal, that is, above 20°, the medial structures will not be able to counteract the excessive lateral force produced and there will be a tendency for the patella to displace laterally (Insall, 1979).

## Bony Factors

Bony factors also exert an influence on the normal tracking of the patella. The lateral condyle of the femur is higher than the medial condyle and this helps to prevent excessive lateral movement of the patella. However, the lateral condyle can be smaller than normal and so predispose the patella to subluxation.

According to Malek and Mangine (1981) the relationship of the vertical size of the patella and the length of the ligamentum patellae should be a 1:1 ratio (Figure 8–3). Variations in this ratio can result in the patella becoming high riding (patella alta) and vulnerable to the pull of the lateral forces, or being positioned lower than usual (patella baja), in which case it is subjected to an increase in compression forces. The patella itself may be smaller than normal, tilted, or oriented too much in a lateral or medial direction; these abnormalities could also contribute to its instability.

## Other Factors Influencing the Lateral Forces on the Patella

James (1979) coined the phrase "miserable malalignment" to describe the angular and torsional malalignments found in the lower extremity of young active people complaining of anterior knee pain. These are:

- an increase in the angle of femoral anteversion;
- excessive internal femoral rotation;
- bilateral squinting patellae (patellae turned inward);
- a genu varum and associated recurvatum;
- increased Q angle;
- external tibial torsion;
- tibial varum;
- foot pronation.

*Note:* There are a number of conditions relating to the patellofemoral joint that develop as a result of abnormal patella tracking

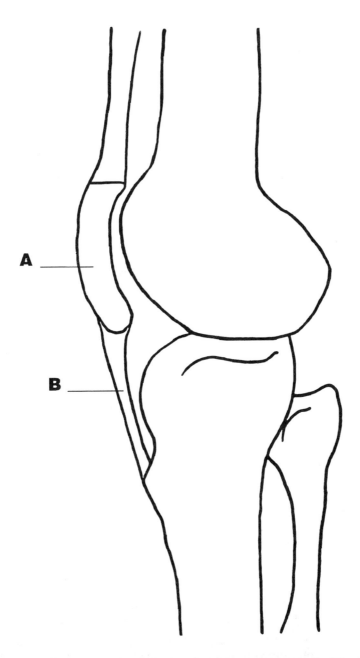

**Figure 8–3.** The 1:1 ratio between the length of the patella (A) and the length of the ligamentum patellae (B) (adapted from Malek & Mangine, 1981).

177

and abnormal patellar compression forces; consequently, it is important to look and test for the presence of the soft tissue and bony abnormalities discussed above when examining any patient complaining of patellofemoral pain.

## MALALIGNMENT SYNDROME

The malalignment syndrome develops as a result of abnormal tracking of the patella; any combination of the factors discussed above can give rise to the syndrome which can be extremely disabling, especially for the athlete.

### Clinical Features

The clinical signs and symptoms listed below are common findings in the malignment syndrome.

- Aching pain may be felt around the knee cap or the medial side of the knee, or sometimes posteriorly, and is aggravated by ascending or descending stairs; it may be experienced in one or both knees and for no apparent reason.
- The pain is made worse by activity and by prolonged sitting (movie sign).
- Patella tenderness is produced with patella compression on the lateral border as attempts are made to passively move the patella medially with the knee flexed over a pillow.
- Midpoint medial tibiofemoral joint line tenderness is a frequent finding, which may confuse the examiner into thinking the problem is attributable to the medial meniscus.
- Other findings that may be present and add to the confusion are joint catching and giving way. The former is probably caused by abnormal tracking of the patella and the latter by inhibition of the quadriceps because of pain (Chen, 1990). These two clinical features are also common in the meniscus injury.

As indicated above there may be some confusion in the examiner's mind because of the elicitation of signs and symptoms that are commonly associated with a meniscus lesion. However, the history of injury or onset, as determined from the assessment, is quite different in the two conditions and differentiation can often be made on this basis.

## Treatment Guidelines

Treatment is dependent on the findings obtained during the assessment procedure.

Rest from repetitive stressful activities with appropriate medication is advocated.

McConnell (1986) focuses on abnormal orientation of the patella in terms of the lateral and rotary components and the tilt, and corrects these; for example, if there is an excessive lateral orientation the following procedures are applied:

- medial glides of the patella to stretch the tight lateral structures;
- application of a specific tape and "undercoat" (skin protector) to pull the patella medially in a pain-free range;
- similarly, if there is an upward or downward tilt of the patella, or the rotary component is emphasized in a medial or lateral direction, this too is corrected by tape;
- with the corrective tape in place eccentric and concentric quadriceps activity in various positions of knee flexion, in the weightbearing position, is introduced.

Kramer (1986) advocates short period of rest and the modality of choice, such as ice and ultrasound, to resolve the symptoms. This is followed by medial displacement of the patella, held for approximately one minute to stretch the tight lateral structures. Isometric quadriceps exercises are performed, initially in extension, followed by isotonic knee extension from the 90° flexed position progressing to full isotonic quadriceps activity.

Abnormal foot pronation is often a significant contributing factor and correction of this can be achieved by the application of the appropriate orthosis.

Several authors, Kramer (1986), Fisher (1986), and Welsh and Hutton (1990a), advocate the use of a patellar brace when the patient returns to activity.

## Surgery

There are numerous surgical approaches that can be used, depending on which particular mechanical fault needs to be corrected. Some of these are listed below:

- lateral retinaculum release;
- proximal realignment of vastus medialis;
- distal realignment of the ligamentum patellae to a more medial location;
- tibial tubercle elevation in conjunction with medial displacement.

All of the above procedures attempt to restore the normal forces acting on the patella, thus eliminating the pain associated with abnormal mechanics. However, conservative treatment of patellofemoral pain has been shown to be effective in the majority of cases (Fisher, 1986; McConnell, 1986; Kramer, 1986).

## CHONDROMALACIA OF THE PATELLA

For many years patellar chondromalacia was thought to be the major cause of patellofemoral pain. Now it is considered by some to be a relatively rare entity (Nofthall, 1990), and the term should be applied only when there is evidence of degeneration (Figure 8–4) to the patellar articular cartilage (Welsh & Hutton, 1990a). Patellar malalignment, as described above, is considered to be the predominant cause of patellofemoral pain and can be a contributing factor in chondromalacia (Insall, 1979).

### The Stages of Degeneration

The degeneration presents itself in four stages (Dandy, 1986; Nofthall, 1990; Outerbridge, 1961).
    The first stage is swelling and softening of the cartilage; fissuring occurs in stage two; there is a breakdown of the cartilage known as fasciculation in stage three; and the final stage is osteoarthritis.
    *Note:* Insall (1979) believes that chondromalacia and osteoarthritis should be regarded as separate entities and Chen (1990) has stated that chondromalacia does not necessarily progress to arthritis.

### Etiology

The condition can develop as a result of:

- patella malalignment;
- recurrent subluxation (see later);

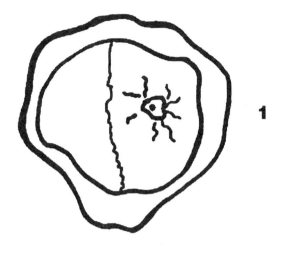

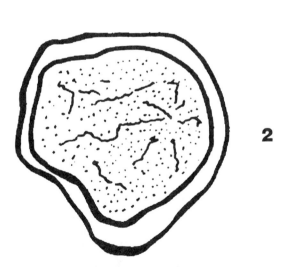

**Figure 8–4.** Chondromalacia of the patella: (1) early stage; and (2) last stage (adapted from Peterson & Renstrom, 1986).

- direct trauma;
- repetitive stress arising from strenuous sporting activities.

## Clinical Features

Some of the same clinical features attributed to the malalignment syndrome are present: for example, patellofemoral pain, giving way, and locking. Other features include:

- crepitus;
- increased pain on patellofemoral compression or because of increased forces on the joint when running, going up and down stairs, or sitting for prolonged periods;
- weakness of the quadriceps;
- tenderness on palpation round the periphery of the patella.

## Treatment

Conservative treatment is tried first for a period of several weeks. This consists of:

- rest from aggravating activities, and ice application;
- if malalignment is thought to be a contributing factor the conservative approach, with focus on the particular malalignment, is tried (see Malalignment Syndrome above);
- anti-inflammatory medication in the form of aspirin has been found to be beneficial in that it is thought to arrest the degradation of the cartilage (Outerbridge & Dunlop,1975);
- strengthening of the quadriceps isometrically then isotonically (Kramer, 1986; McConnell, 1986);
- use of a brace when returning to normal activities.

The surgical approaches (see Malalignment Syndrome) are dependent upon the contributing factor. In addition, patellar shaving has met with some success.

*Note:* As stated previously, for many years patellofemoral pain was thought to be caused by chondromalacia patellae. Conservative treatment in terms of rest, ice, medication, and quadriceps strengthening would sometimes be successful, but often surgery was performed with dubious results. The focus on malalignment and patellar compression forces as causes of patellofemoral pain changed the whole approach to treatment and, as indicated above, these forces can be contributing factors in the development of chondromalacia patellae.

## PATELLAR SUBLUXATION AND DISLOCATION

Patellar subluxation and dislocation occur frequently in athletes (Brown, 1990). Subluxation occurs as a result of an unstable patella arising from abnormal small size, patella alta, and/or excessive lateral forces. Dislocation is usually traumatic in origin, often caused by a violent impact on the medial aspect of the patella, but instability and excessive lateral forces can be predisposing factors. Both injuries can occur when the athlete changes direction.

In subluxation the patella displaces laterally, but not completely so, and then returns to its original position. The patient is aware of the instability and becomes apprehensive if attempts are made to passively displace the patella laterally (the apprehension sign).

Dislocation occurs when the patella is completely displaced laterally and is often accompanied by extensive soft tissue damage to the medial structures. Reduction can occur spontaneously. It can be an isolated incident or recurrent in nature.

### Clinical Features

The clinical features of dislocation are an extension of those found in subluxation. Signs and symptoms relating to soft tissue damage are more prevalent in dislocation:

- anteromedial or parapatellar pain;
- tenderness on palpation of the periphery of the patella, particularly the medial aspect and soft tissue structures;
- effusion (subluxation) or hemarthrosis (dislocation);
- impairment in function (largely caused by apprehension with subluxation and soft tissue damage with dislocation);
- marked quadriceps atrophy after acute dislocation.

### Treatment Guidelines

The focus of treatment for subluxation relates to the limb alignment and foot mechanics:

- ice, compression bandage (if swelling is present);
- strengthening of the quadriceps (particularly vastus medialis) and hamstrings;
- stretching exercises for the lateral retinaculum and iliotibial band;
- orthotic foot support to counteract the effect of excessive pronation or genu valgum;
- patellar brace.

The focus of treatment for a dislocation is to determine the extent of the soft tissue damage and to determine if there are loose bodies present in the joint. The joint is aspirated and surgery is performed to repair or tighten soft tissue structures or to remove loose bodies. This may be followed by the application of a stove pipe cast for approximately four weeks, during which time quadriceps strengthening exercises are instituted. Following removal of the cast, strengthening exercises to hamstrings and quadriceps muscles and exercises to restore full extensibility of the muscle groups become the focus.

# RECURRENT DISLOCATION OF THE PATELLA

Recurrent dislocation of the patella involves episodes of dislocation rather than an isolated incident.

## Causes

Any of the following factors may contribute to this disorder:

- failure of development of the lateral condyle;
- patella situated abnormally high (patella alta);
- general joint laxity;
- abnormal band of fascia leading from the lateral border of the patella to the deep surface of the iliotibial band; the iliotibial band, which moves backwards during flexion, pulls the patella backwards and laterally;
- tightness of the lateral retinaculum or slackness of the medial retinaculum.

## Treatment

Treatment usually involves surgery; some of the procedures used are listed under the treatment for the Malalignment Syndrome.

# JUMPER'S KNEE

Jumper's knee is a tendinitis of the patellar tendon at its attachment to the inferior pole of the patella and is one of the overuse injuries. It develops in athletic sports in which jumping plays an integral role, for example, basketball. Less commonly it is found as a result of lifting excessive weights with the quadriceps.

## Clinical Features

- Pain is experienced in the patellar tendon, increasing on activities that stress the tendon.
- There is tenderness on palpation at the inferior pole of the patella.
- Local swelling may be present.
- An extensor lag may be present.
- Resisted knee extension may increase the pain and will produce a weak result.

## Treatment

The condition responds well to a conservative approach.

- Warm-up exercises and ice are recommended.
- Anti-inflammatory medication may be effective.
- Transverse frictions help to stimulate connective tissue formation and orientation in a normal pattern.
- A tensor bandage will help to counteract some of the forces being transmitted to the tendon.
- Eccentric exercises have been proved very effective (Curwin & Stanish, 1984).

# PATELLAR TENDON RUPTURE

If, in the presence of a jumper's knee, the pain is ignored and more stress is applied to the knee, the tendon may rupture. It is also likely to rupture as a result of excessive loading without existing pathology, for example, when there is a powerful contracture of the quadriceps to counteract the weight of the body applied to the lower extremity (Siwek, 1990).

## Clinical Features

- The knee gives way and the patient falls.
- Close observation reveals that the patella on the affected side rides more proximally than the one on the unaffected side.
- When the knee is flexed the patella does not move inferiorly.
- A palpable gap may exist.
- The injury may be accompanied by an avulsion fracture of the inferior pole of the patella or at the tibial tubercle.

## Treatment

Surgical repair is performed followed by immobilization in extension for 4–6 weeks. At the end of the immobilization period rehabilitation restores range and strength.

## PREPATELLAR BURSITIS (HOUSEMAID'S KNEE) AND INFRAPATELLAR BURSITIS

There are a number of bursae associated with the knee complex (Figure 8–5); the two listed above are intimately related to the patellofemoral joint.

The prepatellar bursa is situated at the front of the knee beneath the skin and overlying the patella. The infrapatellar bursa is located between the ligamentum patellae and the tibia. Their purpose is to eliminate friction. Bursitis can be either acute or chronic.

## Etiology

The conditions develop as a result of a blow or fall directly on the bursa or they can be caused by chronic irritation.

## Clinical Features

- Swelling is present and there is tenderness on palpation.
- Active or passive knee flexion will increase the pain.
- There may be an increase in temperature.

## Treatment Guidelines

The following conservative approaches may be of value:

- ice, compression;
- anti-inflammatory drugs;
- ultrasound;
- quadriceps strengthening and range of motion exercises as swelling decreases.

## FAT PAD SYNDROME (HOFFA'S SYNDROME)

Both the infrapatellar fat pad (Figure 8–5) and the synovium (which is separated from the ligamentum patellae by the infrapatellar fat pad) can become compressed between the patella, or associated soft tissue structures, and the femoral condyles.

## Mechanism of Injury

Acute compression of the fat pad or the synovium usually occurs with sudden forced extension of the knee; chronic syndromes are related to a repetitive activity rather than a history of trauma. In the chronic form, hypertrophy of the synovium and fat pad occurs because of repetitive activity; compression develops and the structures are continually irritated, resulting in persistent symptoms. The fat pad syndrome often develops after arthroscopy or ACL reconstruction using the patellar tendon.

## Clinical Features

- Tenderness is found on palpation of the inferior aspect of the patella.
- The patient complains of pain in the region of the inferior aspect of the patella.
- Swelling may be present.
- Crepitus may be apparent.

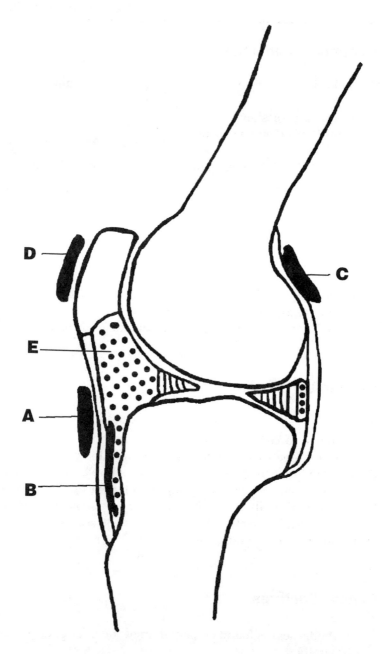

**Figure 8–5.** Bursae around the knee joint and the infrapatellar fat pad: (A) the superficial infrapatellar bursa; (B) the deep (subtendinous) infrapatellar bursa; (C) the lateral gastrocnemcius bursa; (D) the prepatellar bursa; and (E) the infrapatellar fat pad (adapted from Netter, 1989).

## Treatment Guidelines

Useful modalities may include:

- ice;
- ultrasound;
- stretching of the quadriceps to reduce compressive loads;
- decrease in regular activity.

## SUMMARY

With the advent of jogging as a popular pastime the incidence of patellofemoral problems has greatly increased. Many of the problems develop as a result of faulty biomechanics and this chapter began with a review of the biomechanical features of the patellofemoral joint. The first condition discussed was that of the Malalignment Syndrome for which biomechanical faults in the lower extremity are responsible. Chrondromalacia of the patella was presented next, followed by Patellar Subluxation and Dislocation. Jumper's Knee is a condition that affects athletes such as basketball players. It is a partial rupture of the patellar tendon at its attachment to the inferior pole of the patella, and can lead to a disabling tendinitis or to a complete rupture. The chapter concluded with the afflictions of two bursae associated with the patella and finally with the Fat Pad Syndrome.

CHAPTER 9

• • • • • • • •

# The Tibiofemoral Joint

The tibiofemoral joint is a modified hinge joint and is the largest synovial joint in the body. The femur and tibia provide long lever arms situated proximally and distally, respectively, to the center of the joint thus predisposing the ligamentous structures and menisci to injury that often results in severe disability; this is particularly so in athletic activities and motor vehicle accidents (Baugher & White,1985).

In order to understand the mechanism of injury and clinical features involved in the injuries of the tibiofemoral joint, a knowledge of the pertinent anatomy is necessary.

## PERTINENT ANATOMY

A consideration of the bony architecture of the tibiofemoral joint reveals that it is formed from the articulation of the convex medial and lateral femoral condyles and the medial and lateral tibial condyles; the latter are somewhat flat. Congruence is facilitated by the medial and lateral menisci situated on their respective tibial condyles. These will be described in more detail later. Although some stability is achieved by the congruence afforded by the bony architecture and the menisci, the main passive stabilizers are the medial and lateral collateral ligaments and the anterior and posterior cruciate ligaments; these will be discussed next.

## THE PASSIVE STABILIZERS

Noyes, Grood, Butler, and Malek (1980) defined functional stability as that which exists in the knee during static and dynamic situations. In both instances active muscles and passive ligament restraints are employed. The passive structures can be further divided into primary and secondary restrainers for each of the four planes of stability, which are medial, lateral, anterior, and posterior. The passive restrainers are described according to Marshall and Baugher (1980) and Baugher and White (1985).

## Medial Stabilizers Against a Valgus Force

A valgus force is one that is applied to the lateral aspect of the joint in such a way that the tibia is abducted and stress is placed on the medial aspect of the knee (Figure 9–1). The prime stabilizer against such a force with the knee in flexion is the superficial medial collateral ligament (MCL) (Baugher & White, 1985). Secondary stabilizers are the posterior oblique ligament (tendinous expansion of the semimembranosus muscle), medial capsule and ligamentous reinforcements, and the anterior cruciate ligament. The next line of defense is the posterior capsule and finally the posterior cruciate ligament which is regarded as a tertiary line of defense. The secondary and tertiary stabilizers function optimally when the joint is in extension.

## Lateral Stabilizers Against a Varus Force

A varus force is one that is applied to the medial aspect of the joint so that the tibia is adducted and stress is placed on the lateral aspect of the knee (Figure 9-2). The prime stabilizing function is shared by several structures. The lateral collateral ligament is considered to be the prime stabilizer but it is closely associated in its stabilizing function with the secondary stabilizers, namely the popliteus arcuate complex (at the posterolateral aspect of the joint) and the anterior cruciate ligament. The posterior cruciate ligament is considered as a tertiary line of defense.

In addition to the ligamentous structures, muscular structures play a role in the defense against the valgus and varus forces. The medial hamstrings contribute to the restraining process on the medial side of the knee and the iliotibial band makes its contribution to restraint on the lateral side of the knee, particularly with the knee in extension.

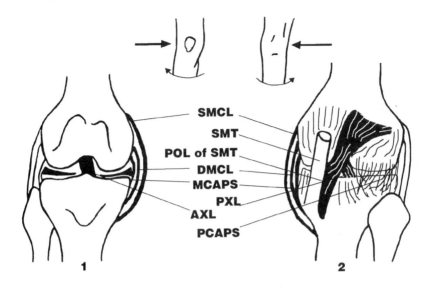

**Figure 9–1.** Stabilizers against a valgus force. Superficial medial collateral ligament (SMCL), semimembranous tendon (SMT), posterior oblique ligament (POL), deep medial collateral ligament (DMCL), medial capsule (MCAPS), posterior cruciate ligament (PXL), anterior cruciate ligament (AXL), and posterior capsule (PCAPS).

The stabilizing structures on the lateral aspect of the joint are not damaged as frequently as the medial stabilizing structures because some protection against a varus force is afforded by the other knee.

## Anterior Tibial Displacement Stabilizers

The prime structure preventing anterior displacement of the tibia on the femur is the anterior cruciate ligament (Figures 9–3 and 9–5). It is also the primary restraint against hyperextension and internal rotation in the almost extended position (Gollehon, Warren, & Wickiewicz, 1985). The secondary stabilizers are the medial and lateral collateral ligaments and associated capsular structures.

## Posterior Tibial Displacement Stabilizers

The prime stabilizer against posterior displacement of the tibia on the femur is the posterior cruciate ligament (Figures 9–4 and 9–5).

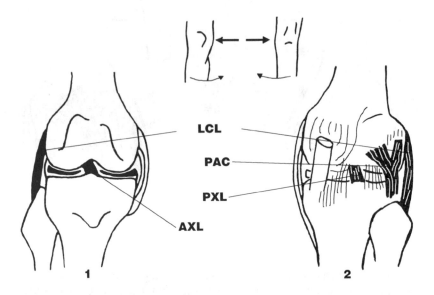

**Figure 9–2.** Stabilizers against a varus force. Lateral collateral ligament (LCL), popliteus arcuate ligament (PAC), posterior cruciate ligament (PXL), and anterior cruciate ligament (AXL).

The secondary stabilizers are the posterior capsule and lateral complex structures.

*Note:* It has been shown that the anterior cruciate ligament (ACL) provides 85 per cent of the restraint during the performance of the anterior drawer test, all other restraints collectively providing 15 per cent. However, in the performance of the anterior drawer test for ACL only a slight laxity may be revealed even in the presence of a complete rupture. This is because only a small force of about 20 pounds is applied which the secondary restrainers are able to counteract. This test is not, therefore, a true predictor of functional stability (Noyes, Grood, Butler, & Malek, 1980). The Lachman test is much more reliable.

## THE MENISCI

The menisci were mentioned briefly before and will now be considered in greater detail. The menisci are fibrocartilaginous structures

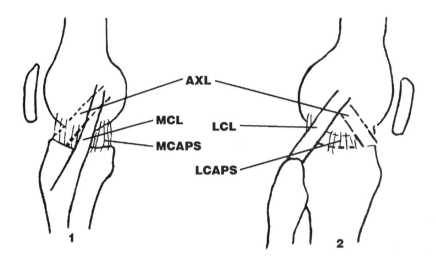

**Figure 9–3.** Stabilizers against anterior tibial displacement. Anterior cruciate ligament (AXL), medial collateral ligament (MCL), medial capsule (MCAPS), lateral collateral ligament (LCL), and lateral capsule (LCAPS).

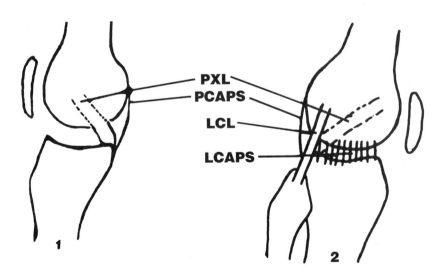

**Figure 9–4.** Stabilizers against posterior tibial displacement. Posterior cruciate ligament (PXL), posterior capsule (PCAPS), lateral collateral ligament (LCL), and lateral capsule (LCAPS).

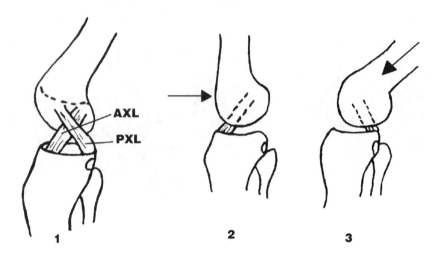

**Figure 9–5.** The cruciate ligaments and their resistance to force. (1) The anterior cruciate ligament (AXL) and the posterior cruciate ligament (PXL). (2) The anterior cruciate ligament resisting a posterior force on the femur. (3) The posterior cruciate ligament resisting an anterior force on the femur (2 & 3 adapted from Basmajian, 1975).

that are semilunar in shape; they have been described in terms of their relationship to a circle (Figure 9–6). The medial meniscus forms a small part of a large circle and the lateral meniscus forms a large part of a small circle. The circles are incomplete at the intercondylar tubercle region of the tibia. Both menisci have an anterior and a posterior horn, which are closer together on the lateral meniscus than the medial meniscus. Each meniscus has three surfaces; the upper surface is concave, the lower surface is somewhat flat, and the periphery is convex. They are wedge shaped in cross section. Except in their peripheral one third and their horns, the menisci are avascular (Mangine & Price, 1988).

## Attachments

The horns of the menisci are attached to the associated areas of the tibial condyles and the anterior horns of both menisci are joined by the **transverse ligament**. The menisci are directly linked to the patella by the fibers that extend from the borders of the patella to the peripheral borders of the menisci; they are known as the **menisco-**

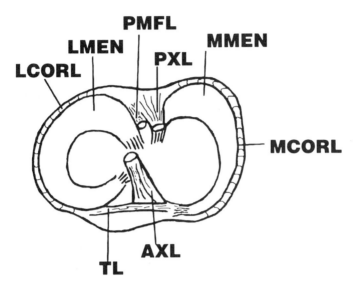

**Figure 9–6.** Superior view of the menisci and associated structures. Anterior cruciate ligament (AXL), medial coronary ligament (MCORL), medial menisus (MMEN), posterior cruciate ligament (PXL), posterior meniscofemoral ligament (PMFL), lateral meniscus (LMEN), lateral coronary ligament (LCORL), and transverse ligament (TL).

**patellar fibers**. There is also an indirect link to the patella through strands extending from the transverse ligament. Both menisci have **capsular attachments** but the attachment on the lateral side is not as extensive as on the medial side.

In addition to the above, the **medial meniscus** is attached to the **MCL** and to the **semimembranosus tendon**; there are also fibers from the **anterior cruciate ligament** inserted into the anterior horn of the meniscus. Finally, there is an extensive attachment to the coronary ligament (Brownstein, Mangine, Noyes, & Kryger, 1988).

The lateral meniscus is a more mobile structure than the medial meniscus; it is not attached to the LCL but it does have attachments at its posterior border to the **popliteus tendon**. It is also attached at its posterior horn to the **posterior cruciate ligament** by fibers which form the **meniscofemoral ligament**.

Obviously the attachments of the menisci to the associated structures described above make them more vulnerable to injury should those structures become traumatized.

## Movements

During flexion and extension of the knee joint the menisci move with the **tibia**. Consequently they will **move backwards during flexion** and **forwards during extension**. This is easy to understand if consideration is given to the attachments of the menisci described above.

During **axial rotation** of the knee the menisci move with the **femoral condyles**. During **lateral rotation of the tibia** the **medial meniscus moves in a posterior direction** and the **lateral meniscus moves in an anterior direction. The reverse occurs during medial rotation of the tibia** (Kapandji, 1987).

## Functions

Apart from increasing the congruence of the knee joint and contributing to the stability, the menisci play an important role in transmission of compressive forces between the femur and tibia. As indicated above they also facilitate smooth movement of the joint.

# CONDITIONS

Additional mechanisms and management of injuries to the ligaments and menisci will be discussed in this section.

## LIGAMENTOUS INJURIES

The manner in which the knee sustained the injury provides a vital lead to diagnosis. The position of the knee, whether it was loaded, and the direction of the applied force, are important factors (Zarins & Nemeth, 1985). Sometimes the patient is unable to provide precise information, but on other occasions the mechanism can be described clearly. However, the examiner must be careful not to jump to a diagnostic conclusion on the basis of the mechanism alone or the clinical findings may be misinterpreted.

## Mechanisms and Their Interpretation

Clancy (1985a) and Zarins and Nemeth (1985) provide useful indicators of injury to the ligaments with and without contact. The mechanisms with contact will be described first.

*Contact Injuries*

**Collateral Ligaments.**  The MCL is injured when a valgus force is applied to the lateral aspect of the leg when the foot is fixed to the ground with the knee in slight flexion (the "clipping injury"). Additional force will rupture the anterior cruciate ligament, since this acts as a secondary restrainer. The LCL is injured if a varus force is applied to the medial aspect of the leg when it is fixed to the ground. However, as stated previously, this is an uncommon injury.

**Cruciate Ligaments.**  If force is applied to the anterior aspect of the extended knee driving it into hyperextension the anterior cruciate ligament will rupture first, but if additional force is applied the posterior cruciate will also be damaged.

Force applied to the anterior aspect of the tibia (when it is in 90° of flexion) as, for example, in a fall on the flexed knee, or a dashboard injury, will result in a torn posterior cruciate.

*Non-contact Injuries*

The most common mechanism of contact injury is that of deceleration, valgus, and external rotation of the leg as occurs when the athlete lands on a slightly flexed knee and turns away from it (Zarins & Nemeth, 1985). Under such circumstances the anterior cruciate will be torn. It has been estimated that 80 per cent of anterior cruciate injuries occur in this manner (Gollehon et al., 1985).

# Location of Pain as an Indicator
# of the Injured Structure

Clancy (1985a) has identified several locations in and around the knee joint where pain can be experienced and has indicated which injured structures are most likely causing the pain.

*Medial Pain*

Pain at the medial joint line, medial femoral condyle, or upper tibia is suggestive of damage to the MCL. Pain at the medial joint line only, could implicate the MCL, the medial meniscus, or the patellofemoral joint.

### Anteromedial or Parapatellar Pain

Anteromedial or parapatellar pain is indicative of a patella subluxation or dislocation. If there has been a dislocation there will always be pain just proximal to the adductor tubercle on the intermuscular septum where the vastus medialis tears from the intermuscular septum.

### Lateral Joint Line Pain

Mid-lateral joint line pain could be caused by a lateral meniscus or a LCL injury. If the pain is also posterolateral a complex meniscus injury must be suspected.

### Posterolateral Pain

Posterolateral pain could be a lateral meniscus injury, but probably it is an avulsion of the anterior cruciate ligament from the femoral condyle. An injury to popliteus may also cause posterolateral pain.

### Posterior Pain

Posterior pain is associated with a mild strain of the gastrocnemius, a mild sprain of the posterior capsule, or a tear of the posterior cruciate ligament.

## COLLATERAL LIGAMENT SPRAINS

There are three degrees of ligamentous sprain; the injury and clinical features of each and treatment guidelines are described below. The MCL is injured more frequently than the LCL and so much of what follows relates to this ligament.

## Injury and Clinical Features

The injury is described first, followed by the clinical features.

### First Degree Sprain (Mild)

In a first degree sprain there is tearing of a minimum number of fibers. The joint surfaces separate 5 mm or less on the affected side.

There is localized tenderness, but no instability. There is a firm end-feel on stress testing.

### Second Degree Sprain (Moderate)

In second degree sprains there is tearing of the maximum number of fibers without producing instability. The joint surfaces separate 5 to 10 mm on the affected side when the knee is stress tested at 30° of flexion but is stable when stress tested in extension.

There is generalized tenderness on the affected side. The patient is unable to bear weight because of the pain. Swelling may be present. A soft end-feel is present with the stress test.

### Third Degree Sprain (Severe)

In third degree sprains there is complete disruption of the ligament with marked instability; the joint surfaces separate 10 mm or more when subjected to the stress test in 30° of flexion. The knee is stable when stress tested in extension.

Pain is not a factor but instability is and there is a very soft end-feel in response to the stress test.

*Note:* If the stress test, applied at 30° of flexion, produces a medial opening this is indicative of damage to the MCL. A stress test in extension which produces a medial opening indicates damage to the MCL and the secondary restraints.

## Conservative Treatment Guidelines

Conservative treatment is the treatment of choice if the damage is confined to the collateral ligament only. The philosophy of the treatment is basically the same regardless of the severity of the sprain. It consists of a progressive program involving strengthening exercises and mobility largely determined by the patient's pain.

- A posterior splint is applied for a week or so and protected weight bearing on crutches is instituted until the patient is able to walk without pain.
- Ice is applied 3 or 4 times during the day in the early stages.
- Quadriceps strengthening exercises begin as soon as possible: quadriceps setting and straight leg raising (SLR).
- Early mobility is gained in the whirlpool or by swimming.

- Straight leg raising against gravity is progressed to SLR working against weights.
- Hamstring and hip strengthening exercises are incorporated into the program.
- The exercise bicycle is recommended when the patient has achieved 90° of knee flexion.
- Isokinetic exercises for the quadriceps are added.
- A running program is commenced when 70 per cent of strength in the quadriceps has been achieved.

The athlete can return to practice when he or she has full range of pain free motion, 90 per cent of the strength of the normal leg, and can complete the running program (Clancy, 1985b).

If incapacitating medial instability persists, the following surgery may be recommended.

## Pes Anserinus Transfer

The pes anserinus is composed of sartorius, gracilis, and semi-tendinosus. The transfer is one of the ancillary procedures used to restore dynamic and static stability to the medial side of the knee. It involves the transfer of the semitendinosus to a more proximal anterior insertion near the patellar tendon (Clancy, 1985b). In so doing the power of medial rotation is enhanced and a sling support (against a valgus thrust) is provided around the medial flare of the tibial condyle (Figure 9–7).

The operation is indicated in the presence of a medial collateral ligament deficiency resulting in increased external rotation of the tibia on the femur. If the procedure is used in isolation, adequate posterior capsular support is necessary for such a transplant to function. If there is posterior laxity the transplant will merely pull the tibia backward rather than providing internal rotation. The transplantation decreases the flexor power of the muscles, but increases significantly the resistance to external rotation of the tibia. Over time, elongation of the muscle tendon may occur reducing the effectiveness of the procedure (Soderberg, 1986).

## CRUCIATE LIGAMENT INJURIES
## A. ANTERIOR CRUCIATE LIGAMENT (ACL)

Injury to the anterior cruciate ligament must be suspected if there is a third degree sprain of the medial collateral ligament. An

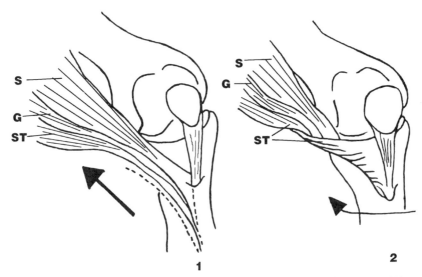

**Figure 9–7.** The pes anserinus transfer. (1) The muscles comprising the pes anserinus: sartorius (S), gracilis (G), and semitendinosus (ST). They act as knee flexors prior to surgery. The dotted lines indicate the surgical incisions that will be made. (2) The pes anserinus acting as a medial rotator following surgery (adapted from Turek, 1984).

arthroscopic examination will either confirm or deny the presence of such an injury. The ligament tears in its middle portion in 80 per cent of patients (Gollehon et al., 1985).

## Mechanism of Injury

An isolated lesion of the anterior cruciate ligament can be the result of a direct contact hyperextension injury sustained when a force is applied to the anterior aspect of the extended knee, especially when the limb is in internal rotation. The lesion may also develop as a result of a non-contact injury as described previously by Zarins and Nemeth (1985).

## Clinical Features

- Rupture of the ligament is usually accompanied by an audible "pop."

- Pain will be present but not necessarily immediately after injury.
- Hemarthrosis develops within two hours and the knee should be aspirated.
- Ability to bear weight will depend upon the integrity of the secondary restrainers.
- There is instability with the knee giving way.
- There is a soft end-feel to anterior displacement of the tibia in response to the Lachman test.

## Treatment Guidelines

The treatment approach selected, namely a conservative approach or a surgical one, is dependent upon the functional demands on the knee following injury. If the secondary restrainers are intact and the anticipated demands on the knee are within the confines of daily activity of a non-athletic nature, a conservative approach focusing upon strengthening of the quadriceps, hamstrings, and associated hip musculature, plus the wearing of a brace at times of additional stress, may be adequate. However, surgery would be the treatment of choice where athletics are a major focus in the patient's life.

## Surgery

Surgical procedures involve intra-articular repair, which is achieved by suturing the two parts of the ligament together, or reconstruction which involves substituting the damaged ligament with another structure such as the semitendinosus tendon or a strip of the patellar tendon. A lateral extra-articular repair in combination with an intra-articular repair may be used (Carson, 1985).

## Rehabilitation

There is no standard treatment protocol following surgical intervention for a damaged anterior cruciate ligament. This is because patients' clinical presentations differ (Engle & Giesen,1991). In most instances it is a long and arduous process. Generally the focus is on allowing sufficient healing time without abnormal stresses. However, the particular approach adopted is dependent on the surgical procedure used and close cooperation between the surgeon and physical therapist. Rehabilitation may follow the lines as advocated by Paulos, Noyes, Grood, and Butler (1981) or be more progressive as advocated by Shelbourne and Nitz (1990). Phasing the rehabilitation program in accordance with the stages of healing and maintenance of function is advocated by Seto, Brewster, Lombardo, and Tibone (1989) and by Reid (1992) in their comprehensive treatment programs.

*Note:* **Sometimes a tear to the anterior cruciate ligament is missed.** Without the implementation of appropriate protective approaches a chronic state develops, in which the secondary restrainers are continually being subjected to stretch thus increasing the instability of the knee joint.

# B. POSTERIOR CRUCIATE LIGAMENT (PCL)

The PCL is the strongest ligament in the knee and is not injured nearly as often as the anterior cruciate ligament, since considerable force is required to disrupt it. It is the prime stabilizer against a posterior displacement of the tibia; this movement is respected during the healing process, therefore hamstring strengthening would be monitored carefully and the emphasis would be on quadriceps strengthening and controlled flexion.

# MENISCUS INJURIES

Meniscus injuries are common knee injuries although not the easiest to diagnose without arthroscopic examination. The medial meniscus is injured more often than the lateral meniscus probably because it is not as mobile and is intimately attached to the medial collateral ligament.

## Mechanism of Injury

External rotation of the foot and lower leg in relation to the femur makes the medial meniscus vulnerable to injury; internal rotation of the foot and lower leg in relation to the femur predisposes the lateral meniscus to injury (Peterson & Renstrom, 1986).

Kapandji (1987) has indicated that the meniscus is vulnerable to injury if it fails to move appropriately with movements of the knee. He gives the following examples:

- Failure of the meniscus to move forward in violent extension of the knee (as in kicking a football) will cause it to become trapped between the femoral and tibial condyles resulting in a transverse tear.
- A twisting movement of the flexed knee causing lateral displacement and lateral rotation (Figure 9–8) forces the medial meniscus to move towards the center of the joint where it will once again be crushed between the condyles when the knee is extended. This mechanism is common in miners and football players and results in a longitudinal tear of the meniscus (bucket handle tear); it can also result in more complex tears.
- Twisting injuries can also result in tears of the anterior and posterior horns (Adams & Hamblen, 1990).

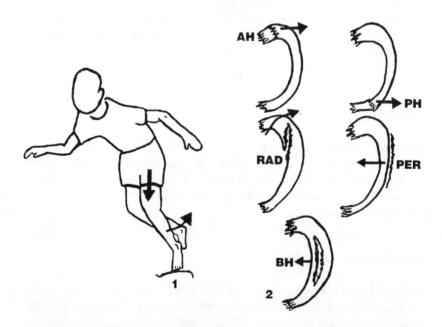

**Figure 9–8.** Mechanism of injury and tears to the medial meniscus. (1) Mechanism of injury (adapted from Helfet, 1974). (2) Tears to the medial meniscus: anterior horn (AH), posterior horn (PH), radial (RAD), peripheral tear (PER), and bucket handle (BH) (adapted from Meade, 1991).

## Clinical Features

The clinical features are similar regardless of the meniscus injured.

- Pain will be experienced on the medial or lateral joint line, depending on which meniscus is injured, particularly on hyperflexion or hyperextension.
- External rotation at 90° of flexion will cause pain in the presence of a medial meniscus problem, and internal rotation at 90° of flexion will cause pain if the lateral meniscus is injured.
- Locking (inability to extend the knee fully) occurs.
- Some effusion may be present.
- There is tenderness on palpation.
- Wasting of the quadriceps develops.

## Surgery

Surgery is performed arthroscopically and can either be a repair for peripheral lesions, which enjoy a high success rate because of the vascularity in the peripheral region, or a partial or complete excision in the avascular region of the meniscus. The partial excision poses more problems for rehabilitation than does the complete excision.

## Post-Surgical Treatment Guidelines

As with the anterior cruciate tear there is no standard approach to treatment. A phased-in approach to rehabilitation for meniscal repair, in accordance with the function and healing rate of the traumatized tissue, is advocated (Mangine & Price, 1988). This involves maximum protection for 3–4 weeks in a hinged brace permitting 30–80°of passive movement, and no weight bearing. Quadriceps and hip exercises, and patellar mobilizations are also part of the program.

The moderate protection phase at the end of 3–4 weeks focuses upon controlled increase in the range of motion, resisted exercises, and gradual weight bearing.

The light activity stage begins between 8–12 weeks after surgery and is concerned with commencing restoration of functional activity. It involves flexibility exercises to all musculature of the lower extremity, isotonic exercises, isokinetic exercises, and endurance activities.

The final stage in the rehabilitation program focuses on returning the patient to full functional activity.

*Note:* Rosenberg and Sherman (1992) have pointed out the importance of the recognition of the high incidence of meniscus injury associated with injury to the anterior cruciate ligament and the implications in terms of establishing a program for management of these patients.

## OSGOOD-SCHLATTER'S DISEASE

Osgood-Schlatter's disease has been described as a tendinitis involving the tibial apophysis (Welsh & Hutton, 1990b). The attachment of the tubercle to the tibia is a weak link in adolescents, usually in boys between the ages of 10 and 15 years. Repeated traction stresses brought on by excessive quadriceps activity pull on the tubercle adversely affecting ossification. It is often a self-limiting disease.

### Signs and Symptoms

The major clinical findings are:

• pain in the region of the tibial tubercle, which is enlarged;
• swelling of the patellar tendon;
• tenderness on pressure over the tubercle.

### Treatment Guidelines

The purpose of the treatment is to reduce the stress on the tibial tubercle by adopting the following approaches:

• decreased athletic activity;
• ice to the tibial tubercle;
• quadriceps stretching;
• static quadriceps exercises progressing to small arc of motion exercises;
• SLR (pain must be minimum).

The above program is progressed to strengthening and activity sessions, but pain must be monitored throughout. In severe cases it may be necessary to immobilize the knee in a plaster cylinder extending from the groin to the malleoli for 6–8 weeks (Adams & Hamblen, 1990).

## OSTEOCHONDRITIS DISSECANS

A portion of necrotic subchondral bone often about 2cm in size (Adams & Hamblen, 1990), develops on the lateral margin of the medial femoral condyle (the most common site) in children or adolescents. An area of demarcation develops around the portion of bone. Although spontaneous healing can occur it is common for a fragment to separate partially or completely from the parent bone and become a loose body in the joint. The cause is unknown although impingement of the tibial spine against the condyle during excessive internal rotation, or circulatory obstruction, have been proposed (Turek, 1984).

### Signs and Symptoms

The signs and symptoms of osteochondritis dissecans are:

- discomfort in the knee which is made worse by exercise;
- swelling which may be present as a result of reaction of the synovium;
- possible locking and "giving way" of the knee;
- wasting of the quadriceps.

### Treatment

The fragment of bone is surgically removed or replaced in position by a pin (Adams & Hamblen, 1990).

## PLICA SYNDROME

Patel (1978) first described the synovial folds inside the knee and later defined plica as a "reduplication of the synovial fold" (Patel, 1986). He has described three such synovial folds, the suprapatellar plica, the medial patellar plica and the infrapatellar plica (Figure 9–9). The medial patellar plica has been identified as the one that is likely to cause symptoms, but the extent is debatable (Broom & Fulkerson, 1986). Irrgang (1988) refers to **"the plica"** and describes it as extending from the undersurface of the vastus lateralis, passing transversely to the medial wall of the medial femoral condyle and then distally and obliquely to attach in the

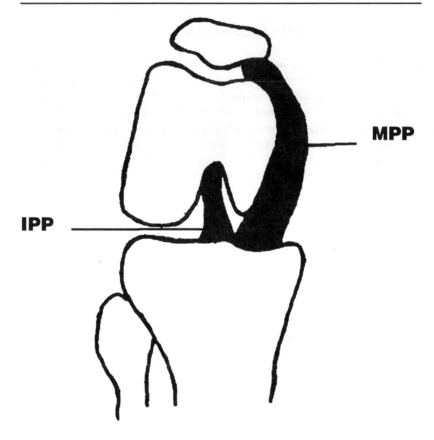

**Figure 9–9.** The medial patellar plica (MPP) and the infrapatellar plica (IPP) (adapted from Patel, 1986).

area of the infrapatellar fat pad. It is present in 20–60 per cent of all knees. It is injured by a direct blow, or by a stretching or tearing caused by a twisting motion or overuse. Inflammation develops with edema and thickening. With overuse it can become a tough fibrotic band.

## Signs and Symptoms

Irrgang (1988) attributes the following clinical features to an injured plica.

- The patient complains of pain medial to the patella that is increased by prolonged sitting (a position that draws the plica tight between the patella and the condyles).

- There is tenderness medial and superior to the patella where the plica can be palpated.
- The plica may snap over the femoral condyle as the knee is flexed and extended.
- There may be a positive "stutter" test: The patient sits over the side of the plinth facing the examiner who places his/her hand on the patella as the knee is actively extended. The patella is seen to jump between 45° and 60° of flexion as it slides over the plica.
- Medial displacement of the patella with the knee at 30° of flexion produces pain.
- The quadriceps are weak and atrophied.
- Tight hamstrings usually exist. This tightness adds to the compression force because the quadriceps are forced to work against shortened hamstrings.

## Treatment Guidelines

Conservative treatment in the form of transverse friction massage over the plica to prevent fibrosis, and exercises to stretch the hamstrings and to strengthen the quadriceps isometrically are advocated by Irrgang (1988). Surgical removal of the plica is the treatment of choice of Patel (1986) and Broom and Fulkerson (1986).

## TRAUMATIC SYNOVITIS (EFFUSION)

Traumatic synovitis is not a diagnosis but an indication of injury to the synovial membrane. It accompanies most acute injuries to the knee joint, but not all. The presence or absence of effusion does not relate to the severity of injury and it is necessary to perform a thorough investigation to determine whether structures other than the synovial membrane have been injured.

## Clinical Features

- Swelling develops usually within six hours of the injury.
- The effusion occupies the horseshoe shape of the suprapatellar pouch.
- The patient complains of discomfort.
- There is no local rise in temperature.

## Treatment Guidelines

If only the synovial membrane has been damaged the treatment is relatively simple:

- rest, ice, compression bandage, to promote absorption;
- isometric quadriceps exercises;
- aspiration which may be necessary if the fluid is present in large quantities.

## TRAUMATIC HEMARTHROSIS (BLOOD IN THE JOINT SPACE)

The swelling of hemarthrosis develops as a result of severe injury to soft tissue structures, commonly the anterior cruciate ligament.

## Clinical Features

- Swelling occurs within a short space of time.
- It is a much more painful condition than synovial effusion.
- There is a thickened consistency compared with effusion which is bouncy.
- There is local temperature increase.

## Treatment Guidelines

Since it has been stated that hemarthrosis accompanies severe injuries it is important that the extent of tissue damage be determined by thorough investigation, under anesthetic if necessary. Aspiration is essential, not only to facilitate the arthroscopic examination process, but also because blood is incompatible with articular cartilage and **causes degenerative changes**. Treatment is then determined by the structure or structures injured.

## ILIOTIBIAL BAND SYNDROME (RUNNER'S SYNDROME)

The iliotibial band is part of the tensor fasciae latae. It extends down the lateral aspect of the thigh and is inserted into Gerdy's tubercle and the lateral tibial condyle. At the level of the knee it divides into the **iliopatellar band** and the **iliotibial band**. The former helps to prevent medial subluxation of the patella and the latter functions as an anterolateral ligament of the knee joint (Terry, Hughston & Norwood, 1986). In the flexed knee the iliotibial band lies posterior to the axis of the knee joint and in extension it lies anterior to the joint (Figure 9–10). Consequently there is a forward and backward motion of the iliotibial band over the epicondyle of the lateral femoral condyle as the knee moves from flexion to extension.

In runners the movement of the band is continuous and the result is an overuse syndrome resulting from friction between the iliotibial band and the lateral femoral epicondyle. Overlying the epicondyle there is a bursa and the resulting problem can be irritation of the band and periosteum and inflammation of the bursa (Renne, 1975). Others have defined the problem simply as a bursitis (Peterson & Renstrom, 1986; Welsh & Hutton, 1990b). The condition is particularly troublesome in runners with a tight iliotibial band or a varus deformity of the knee (Irrgang, 1988).

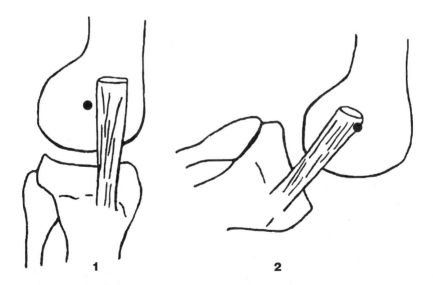

**Figure 9–10.** Relationship of the iliotibia l band to the axis of the knee joint. (1) With the knee in extension the band lies anterior to the axis. (2) In knee flexion the band lies posterior to the axis of the knee joint.

## Clinical Features

The clinical features are consistent with either an inflammation of the iliotibial band and/or a bursitis:

- Pain over the lateral femoral epicondyle, which may be sudden in onset, may quickly incapacitate the runner; the pain ceases when running is discontinued, but returns on resumption of running.
- There is point tenderness above the joint line over the lateral epicondyle.

## Treatment Guidelines

Guidelines for treatment are the same as for any overuse activity. The acute symptoms are treated and the overuse state is avoided by adhering to appropriate training principles.

- The patient is advised to decrease activity and not run beyond the threshold of pain.
- Ice is applied as well as stretching to the iliotibial band.
- Re-education is provided in training techniques with regard to distance and type of surface on which the running takes place.
- Orthotics are useful.

## MUSCLE STRAINS AND HEMATOMAS

Muscle strains and associated hematomas are common injuries in athletes. They can be caused by an intrinsic mechanism, either by overstretching (or overuse) by the athlete, or by compression. The latter usually involves contact with another player such that the muscle is compressed against the bone with resultant tearing (Peterson & Renstrom, 1986). There are three grades of muscle strain and these are described below.

*Grade 1.* When caused by distraction as, for example, in a sudden eccentric muscle activity, a "pulled muscle" results in which the limit of the muscle elasticity is reached but not exceeded (Krejci & Koch,1979). Lachman (1988) and Peterson and Renstrom (1986) feel that in a Grade 1 strain a small percentage of muscle fibers can be torn.

*Grade 2.* In this injury fibers are torn but it is still a partial muscle tear. A hematoma can develop at the site of the injury because retraction of the muscle fibers occurs resulting in a slight depression which fills with blood.

*Grade 3.* This is a complete rupture of the muscle caused by the mechanisms described previously. Retraction of the ends of the muscle fibers occurs resulting in a visible lump.

## Clinical Features

The clinical features will vary in accordance with the type of strain.

- The injury occurs suddenly, accompanied by severe pain and tenderness.
- The patient is unable to use the affected muscle because of pain.
- A palpable and visible depression or gap occurs in Grades 2 and 3 injuries, but this may be eliminated as blood fills the gap.
- Bruising and swelling are visible in Grade 2, and the muscle fibers may be seen to bunch in Grade 3.
- Attempts to contract the muscle will not produce active movement in Grade 3.

## Treatment Guidelines

Treatment guidelines will differ depending upon the extent of the injury. Generally speaking the aims are to decrease pain, to control the hematoma since it delays healing, to control activity in accordance with pain, and to minimize the area of scar tissue. These are achieved in the following ways:

- rest, ice packs, compression bandage, and adhesive bandage;
- anti-inflammatory drugs;
- ultrasound;
- graduated static exercises and dynamic exercises to the threshold of pain;
- stretching exercises;
- massage;
- proprioceptive exercises and resumption of training.

*Note:* It must be remembered that recently formed scar tissue is highly vascular and if stretched can tear easily resulting in more hemorrhage and inflammation. At the same time **complete** rest is not advisable for muscle injuries because atrophy will occur and the scar will contract (Lachman, 1988).

## SUMMARY

The tibiofemoral joint is particularly prone to injury because of its vulnerability in the flexed position. This chapter began with a discussion relating to passive stabilizers (the ligamentous structures) of the joint against a variety of forces. An attempt was made to identify these structures in their roles as primary and secondary restrainers. Next the movements of the menisci were described in relation to the movements of the tibiofemoral joint. Conditions were discussed in which injuries were sustained to the collateral ligaments, the cruciate ligaments, and the menisci respectively. Osgood-Schlatter's disease, a condition affecting the tibial tubercle, was described next, followed by Osteochondritis Dissecans. A less well known entity, the Plica Syndrome, followed by Traumatic Synovitis and Hemarthrosis completed this section of the problems affecting the tibiofemoral joint. The Iliotibial Band Syndrome, another common condition affecting athletes, and a discussion relating to Muscle Strains and Hematomas completed the chapter.

CHAPTER 10

• • • • • • • • •

# The Ankle and Foot

The ankle and foot present a series of inter-related and inter-dependent joints (Figure 10–1) in which an injury sustained by one joint can influence the function of the others. Consequently a knowledge of the pertinent anatomy and biomechanical principles provides a useful background from which to study injuries in this region.

## PERTINENT ANATOMY AND BIOMECHANICAL PRINCIPLES

Knowledge in the area of ankle and foot anatomy and biomechanics is complex, often confusing, and sometimes conflicting. What follows is a simplified approach that will hopefully give the reader an idea of the stabilizing factors, interrelationships between the ankle joint, the subtalar joint, and the transverse tarsal joint, and the relationship of all three to the transverse rotations of the leg.

The joints of the ankle and foot consist of:

- the ankle, or talocrural joint,
- the subtalar joint,
- the transverse tarsal joint,
- the tarsometatarsal joints, and
- the metatarsophalangeal joints.

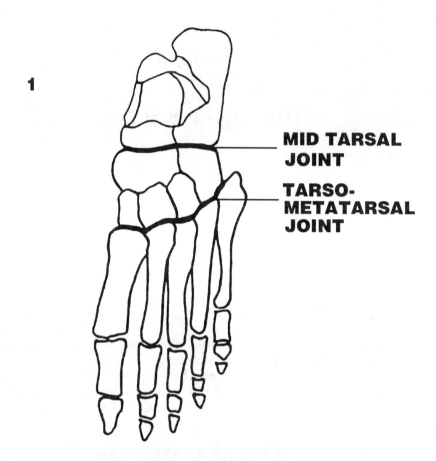

**1**

MID TARSAL
JOINT

TARSO-
METATARSAL
JOINT

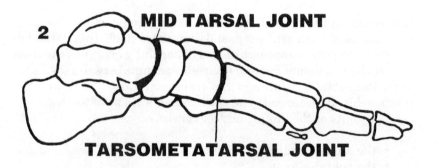

MID TARSAL JOINT

**2**

TARSOMETATARSAL JOINT

**Figure 10–1.** Major joints of the foot as shown (1) from the dorsal aspect and (2) from the medial aspect.

# ANKLE JOINT

Kapandji (1987) has described the ankle joint as being formed from the following articulations:

- the concave inferior tibial surface with the convex superior surface (the trochlear surface) of the talus;
- the medial surface of the talus, which is almost plane, with the lateral surface of the medial malleolus;
- the concave lateral surface of the talus with the facet on the medial surface of the lateral malleolus.

Consideration of the above articulations reveals that the inferior surfaces of the tibia and the corresponding surfaces of the medial and lateral malleoli form a mortise which embraces the trochlea of the talus.

The stability of the ankle joint in the weightbearing position is contributed to by the congruence of the articular surfaces described above, ligamentous support, and associated muscle activity. In addition, the position assumed by the ankle at the time of stress influences stability (Donatelli, 1990). Stormont, Morrey, An, and Cass (1985) have shown that in the weightbearing ankle the articular surfaces are responsible for 30 per cent of the stability relating to rotation and 100 per cent of the stability relating to inversion and eversion. The ankle has the greatest stability in the close packed position of dorsiflexion and is most vulnerable in the loose packed position of plantar flexion.

## Medial Ligamentous Structures

The medial ligamentous structures (Figure 10–2 diagram 1) provide more stability than do the lateral ligamentous structures (Moore, 1980) and provide protection against a valgus or eversion force. Injury to these structures occurs much less often than to the lateral ligamentous structures. The primary ligament on the medial side is the **deltoid ligament**, which is a strong triangular structure arising from the anterior and posterior aspects of the tibial malleolus and from its apex. Netter (1989) divides the ligament into four parts for the purpose of description; these are:

- the posterior tibiotalar ligament;
- the tibiocalcanean ligament;

- the tibionavicular ligament;
- the anterior tibiotalar ligament.

## Lateral Ligamentous Structures

The ligamentous support on the lateral side is not as strong as the medial side and, so is more easily injured during inversion type sprains. The main ligamentous support is provided by the **lateral collateral ligament** (Figure 10–2 diagram 2), which is composed of three ligaments. Because of the frequency of injury to the lateral ligament complex these will be described functionally.

- The anterior talofibular ligament, whose fibers are almost vertical in plantar flexion, acts to restrain the talus during this movement.
- The calcaneofibular ligament prevents the calcaneum and talus from inverting during a varus stress. This ligament is much stronger than the anterior talofibular ligament.
- The posterior talofibular ligament is the strongest of the three; it functions to restrain dorsiflexion. It is rarely injured.

The lateral malleolus, which is larger and extends distally further than the medial malleolus, is considered to be the main restraining structure to lateral talar shifts (Donatelli, 1990). However, it can be fractured in a severe sprain of the medial ligamentous structures.

## SUBTALAR JOINT

The subtalar joint is formed by the articulation of the talus on the calcaneum. It has been described as an oblique hinge that translates the transverse rotation of the lower extremity (external or internal rotation) to inversion or eversion of the calcaneum respectively (Mann, Baxter, & Lutter, 1981; Donatelli, 1990). In addition, the subtalar joint influences the stability of the mid-tarsal joint and the forefoot. Calcaneal inversion increases the stability of the mid-tarsal joint and the forefoot, and eversion reduces the stability. If this is applied to the gait pattern it will be seen that immediately following heel contact, to the foot flat position, the tibia goes into internal rotation, the calcaneum goes into eversion, and the foot is pronated. This is the loose packed position of the foot and enables

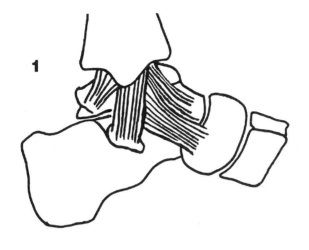

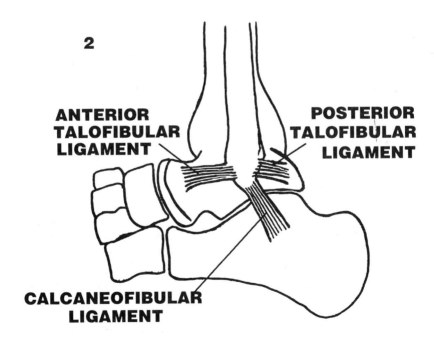

**ANTERIOR TALOFIBULAR LIGAMENT**

**POSTERIOR TALOFIBULAR LIGAMENT**

**CALCANEOFIBULAR LIGAMENT**

**Figure 10–2.** The collateral ligaments of the ankle joint. The medial collateral ligament (1) and the component parts of the lateral collateral ligament (2).

it to be a more efficient shock absorber and to more readily adjust to the ground surface. The foot becomes close packed at the mid-stance phase in gait to the toe off phase. Here it can be seen that the leg goes into external rotation, the calcaneum is inverted, and the foot is supinated providing a rigid lever (Mann et al., 1981).

The relationship between the transverse rotations of the leg and the subsequent movement of the foot can readily be observed in the standing position. If the trunk is rotated to the left it will be seen that the right leg internally rotates, the foot pronates, and the calcaneum everts; the reverse is the case with the left leg and foot.

## MID-TARSAL JOINT (TRANSVERSE TARSAL JOINT)

The mid-tarsal joint is formed from the articulations of the talus and the navicular on the medial side of the foot and the calcaneum and cuboid on the lateral side. Because of their similarity in function the two joints are usually considered together (Soderberg, 1986). It was mentioned earlier that the transverse tarsal joint is influenced by movement of the subtalar joint. This is because, as the subtalar joint moves in a given direction, it appears to pull the transverse tarsal joint in the same direction. When the calcaneum becomes inverted in supination of the foot it pulls the transverse tarsal joint with it, providing more stability. The reverse happens with eversion occurring in pronation (Oatis, 1988).

*Note:* Oatis (1988) feels that because of the complexity of the axes associated with movements of the ankle and foot, movements cannot be described in terms of the cardinal planes with perpendicular axes. She feels it is more appropriate to consider the movements of the joints of the ankle and foot as being triplanar motions because the axes are not perpendicular to the planes of motion and movement is not confined to one plane. Oatis recommends that these triplanar motions be described in terms of pronation (dorsiflexion, abduction, and eversion) and supination (plantarflexion, adduction, and inversion). Consequently the components of these triplanar motions are present in the movements of the three joints discussed above, albeit to different degrees.

## CONDITIONS

Because of the increase in involvement in physical activity and, in particular, competitive athletic activities, the foot and ankle have been subjected to greater stress and trauma. Much of this stress and trauma have had their effect on the structures around the heel. The major predisposing factor is inadequate training methods that result in overuse of these soft tissue structures. Even with adequate training methods the reality is that not everybody is biomechanically perfect, and this factor, in conjunction with the superincumbent weight, creates additional problems. The following conditions are among the most common affecting the foot and ankle.

## LATERAL LIGAMENT SPRAIN

It has been stated that sprain of the lateral ligament is the most common injury in sports (Lassiter, Malone, & Garrett, 1989; McPoil & McGarvey, 1988). Earlier in this chapter the component parts of the lateral ligament (collateral ligament) were reviewed and it was found that this ligament is weaker than its partner on the medial side. The injury sustained is classified in a similar way to muscle strains, in that there are three different grades of injury. These will be described later along with their clinical features.

## Mechanism of Injury

The injury is usually sustained when landing on a plantarflexed and inverted foot from a jump, or when running (Lassiter et al., 1989). Others feel it is a straight inversion sprain (Clanton, 1989; Costello, 1990; McPoil & McGarvey, 1988). Oatis (1988) would describe it as a supination injury. In the plantar flexed position and inverted position the anterior talofibular ligament is subjected to the greatest stress and is likely to tear. As the foot turns inwards, during inversion, the stress is placed on the calcaneofibular ligament and tearing of this ligament occurs. If the tearing is complete there will be a positive anterior drawer test in the first instance, and, in the second instance, there will be a positive lateral stability test.

## Clinical Features Related to the Grade of Injury

The clinical features have been well described in the literature and what follows is a summary.

### Grade 1 Sprain

Grade 1 is a mild sprain resulting in tearing of a few fibers of the anterior talofibular and possibly the calcaneofibular ligaments. The anterior talofibular ligament is primarily affected and the following clinical features are present:

- there is minimum swelling and tenderness about the lateral malleolus;
- some bruising is present;
- pain is felt on stress testing but there is no instability present;
- the patient is able to bear weight with some discomfort;
- there is some loss of range of motion.

### Grade 2 Sprain

Grade 2 is a more severe sprain in which both the anterior talofibular and the calcaneofibular ligaments are involved; the ligamentous tearing is extensive and may be almost complete. The following clinical features are present:

- moderate pain and swelling;
- bruising is extensive, usually distal to the malleolus;
- the patient has difficulty in weight bearing because of pain;
- there is some loss of range of motion;
- instability, if present, is slight.

### Grade 3 Sprain

In grade 3 sprain there is complete ligamentous disruption. The following clinical features are present:

- marked swelling, tenderness, bruising and pain;
- inability to bear weight;
- considerable loss of range of motion;
- positive stability tests.

## Treatment Guidelines

There is general agreement on the treatment approaches for grades 1 and 2 sprains. The aims are to control the extent of the injury, to bring about early restoration of movement, and to return the patient to his or her former activity level. The following approach is recommended by Costello (1990).

- rest, ice, compression, and elevation for the first 24–72 hours;
- early mobility exercises in terms of dorsiflexion and plantarflexion, isometrics, progressing to all movements as tolerated;
- strapping;
- weightbearing without crutches for a Grade 1 sprain and with crutches for a Grade 2 sprain in accordance with pain tolerance;
- increase in the range and strength of all movements; the peronei require particular attention;
- proprioceptive exercises (wobble board);
- restoration of all functional activities.

Grade 3 sprains are those that exhibit varying degrees of instability. If only the anterior talofibular ligament is ruptured there will be a forward subluxation of the talus; if the calcaneofibular ligament is also ruptured there will be varus instability as well. A conservative approach to treatment involving immobilization in a below knee plaster cast may be considered for older people. In younger athletic patients primary surgical repair would be the treatment of choice (Hutton, 1985). Following surgical repair Costello (1990) recommends application of a plaster cast for about ten days followed by the application of a functional splint for six weeks which permits some movement in the sagittal plane. When the splint is removed the rehabilitation program progresses along the lines outlined for a Grade 2 sprain.

*Note:* Hagmeyer and Van Der Wurff (1987) have pointed out that transchondral fractures of the talus can accompany lateral ligament sprains and are often overlooked. They feel that early detection of these fractures is imperative if a successful treatment regimen is to be implemented.

## HEEL PAIN

There are many conditions that give rise to pain in and around the heel. They have been classified by Doxey (1987) and by Adams and Hamblen (1990); they are described below in terms of their location.

## POSTERIOR HEEL PAIN

A common cause of posterior heel pain arises from indirect trauma to the **tendo achilles**. The trauma results in Achilles tendinitis or rupture of the tendo achilles. Other causes of posterior heel pain are **retrocalcaneal bursitis** and, less commonly **tendoachilles bursitis and calcaneal apophysitis (Sever's disease)**.

## A. ACHILLES TENDINITIS AND RUPTURE OF THE ACHILLES TENDON

Achilles tendinitis is a common injury, particularly in the middle aged athlete. The Achilles tendon is not enclosed in a sheath, as other tendons are, such as the peronei; instead it is contained within a highly vascular loose connective tissue called the peritenon (Adams & Hamblen, 1990). The tendon receives its blood supply from two different sources, a proximal supply from the muscle and a distal supply from the calcaneum; the peritenon is likely to have an inflammatory response to minor trauma (Welsh & Huffer, 1990). The combined blood supply meets at a level about 2–3 cm above the insertion of the tendon, where an area of avascularity is created because of the stretching and compression forces to which the tendon is subjected during movement. (It will be recalled that a similar area of avascularity is present in the supraspinatus tendon in the rotator cuff, but not for the same reason.) The area of avascularity may make the tendon susceptible to degeneration. Consequently, the Achilles tendon is vulnerable to injury from two aspects—the inflammatory response from the peritenon, and the degenerative reaction from the area of avascularity.

Rupture of the tendon may be preceded by degeneration but it can occur in isolation in healthy tendons.

### Mechanism of Injury

The inflammatory and degenerative states are overuse injuries seen in runners and are usually attributable to such factors as excessive mileage and inappropriate footwear. Clement, Taunton, and Smart (1984) have suggested that lack of flexibility in the soleus-gastrocnemius complex and excessive pronation are also contributing factors.

Rupture of the tendon occurs unexpectedly and suddenly. Sullivan (1990) describes the mechanism of injury as a sudden change of direction when the runner is decelerating or retreating, or when the ankle is changing from dorsiflexion to plantarflexion in a full weightbearing position; these stresses cause the contracting calf muscles to sustain additional loading.

## Clinical Features

The injury will present itself as an acute inflammatory reaction affecting the tendon and/or the peritenon, or a degenerate response of slow onset, or a complete rupture.

- Pain at the attachment of the tendon or above it, which increases with activity, is usually the symptom that causes the patient to seek help. It may be intermittent, occurring at the early part of the run, or it develops slowly and then persists. If a rupture has occurred the patient will feel as if he or she has sustained a sharp blow about 2–6 cm above the insertion of the tendon.
- There is tenderness on palpation of the tendon and/or the peritenon.
- Thickening of the tendon may be palpable.
- The patient walks with a limp.
- Crepitus is often present.
- There is an inability to walk on the toes if a rupture has occurred.
- Immediately after the rupture has occurred a palpable gap is evident that will quickly become filled with fluid.

## Conservative Treatment Guidelines for Achilles Tendinitis

An effective program may include, as indicated, rest, ice, anti-inflammatory drugs, ultrasound, stretching exercises for the gastrocnemius and soleus, strengthening exercises, use of an appropriate orthotic device to correct any biomechanical problem, and correction of training errors. Curwin and Stanish (1984) have had considerable success with their treatment of Achilles tendinitis, which includes most of the above, but which also focuses on an eccentric exercise program for gastrocnemius and soleus.

## Surgery

The torn ends of the tendon are sutured together with the foot in plantar flexion, followed by immobilization in a cast for about 6 weeks.

## B. RETROCALCANEAL AND TENDOACHILLES BURSITIS

There are two bursae situated on the posterior aspect of the heel (Figure 10–3). The retrocalcaneal bursa lies between the Achilles tendon and the posterior tuberosity of the calcaneum; it is always present. The tendoachilles bursa is more superficial; it lies within the subcutaneous tissue and adjacent to the tendoachilles insertion. It is considered to be adventitious in nature and is not always present (Turek, 1984).

### Clinical Features of Retrocalcaneal Bursitis

- Men are more commonly affected than women.
- Swelling is present where the bursa is located.
- Pain can be elicited by squeezing the tissues just anterior to the tendoachilles.
- The pain is diffuse in nature and is aggravated by dorsiflexion.

### Clinical Features of Tendoachilles Bursitis

- The condition is found only in women.
- There is redness and swelling at the back of the heel on a level with the upper part of the shoe counter (the counter is the part of the shoe that embraces the heel).
- The skin is rough and fissured.

### Treatment Guidelines

Posterior pressure on the heel should be eliminated; consequently footwear which incorporates this principle, such as mules, could be worn temporarily. An elevated heel would take the stretch off the tendoachilles and thus reduce symptoms and further trauma. When the symptoms subside advice regarding appropriate footwear is mandatory.

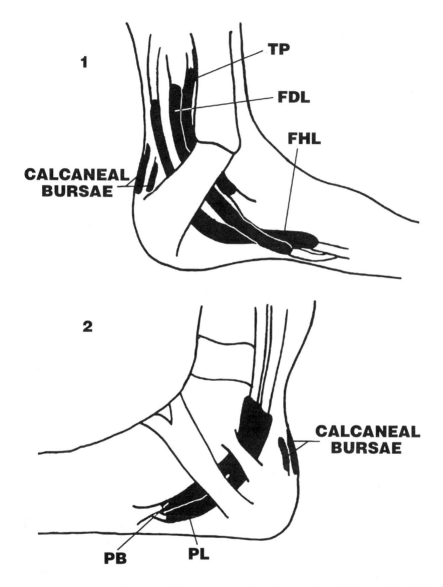

**Figure 10–3.** Calcaneal bursae and tendons about the ankle. (1) The medial aspect of ankle and foot showing the tendons of tibialis posterior (TP), flexor digitorum longus (FDL), and flexor hallucis longus (FHL). (2) The lateral aspect of the ankle and foot showing the tendons of peroneus brevis (PB) and peroneus longus (PL).

## C. CALCANEAL APOPHYSITIS (SEVER'S DISEASE)

The cause of calcaneal apophysitis is strain of the posterior apophysis (growth center), where it attaches to the calcaneum, producing an inflammatory reaction. It occurs only in children during their growth years. The condition is similar to Osgood-Schlatter's disease of the tibial tubercle.

### Mechanism of Injury

The mechanism of injury is thought to arise from the pull of the Achilles tendon on the apophysis at the lower part of the posterior aspect of the heel.

### Clinical Features

The child will complain of pain over the apophysis which will be tender on palpation. Because of the discomfort the child may limp.

### Treatment Guidelines

With rest from activities that involve excessive use of the calf muscles, the condition usually subsides.

## INFERIOR HEEL PAIN

Pain beneath the heel is a very common and disabling symptom. The most common condition arising in this area is **plantar fasciitis** and its often associated condition **calcaneal spur**. Another cause of inferior heel pain is the **medial tarsal tunnel syndrome**, which is a compression neuropathy; pain can also develop from the **heel pad**.

## A. PLANTAR FASCIITIS

Plantar fasciitis is a chronic inflammatory condition affecting the plantar fascia of the foot. In order to appreciate the clinical manifestations of this condition a quick review of the anatomy of this structure will be helpful.

## Pertinent Anatomy

The plantar fascia (Figure 10–4) arises from the medial process of the calcaneal tuberosity on the sole of the foot. The thickest portion is the central portion that divides into five processes at the level of the heads of the metatarsals. Each process has a superficial portion, inserting into the skin, and a deep portion that divides into two slips inserting into either side of the flexor tendons (Warwick & Williams, 1973). The plantar fascia provides support to the sole of the foot and particularly to the medial longitudinal arch. As weight is borne on the foot the two attachments of the plantar fascia are separated and the plantar fascia tightens. In the heel off phase of gait it functions like a windlass (Figure 10–5) providing additional stability to the medial longitudinal arch (Nordin & Frankel, 1989).

## Etiology

The cause of this condition is not thoroughly understood, but in the athlete, it is likely to be caused by repetitive stress, at the attachment of the fascia to the calcaneum ( Doxey, 1987; Welsh & Huffer, 1990). The repetitive stress, in conjunction with biomechanical problems, such as excessive pronation, causes an inflammatory reaction in the plantar fascia, particularly at its insertion into the medial process on the calcaneal tuberosity (Doxey, 1987; Kosmahl & Kosmahl, 1987). The repetitive stresses will cause remodelling of the bone, in order to withstand the stress, with the result that a calcaneal spur is often found in relationship to plantar fasciitis. Torg (1990) feels that the inflammatory process could be caused by restriction of motion in dorsiflexion as a result of a tight gastrocnemius and soleus.

## Clinical Features

The most common symptom is pain beneath the heel at the point of attachment of the plantar fascia. Other clinical manifestations are evident.

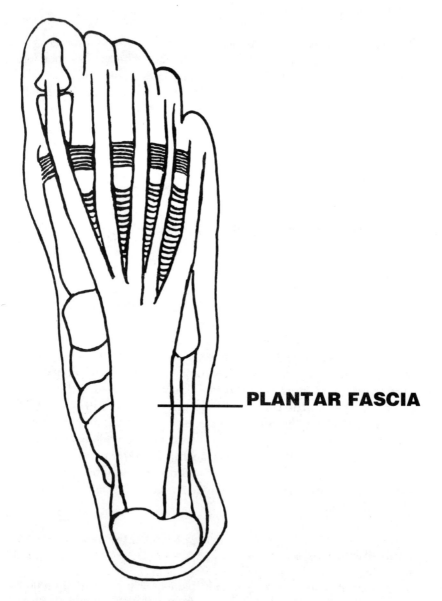

**PLANTAR FASCIA**

**Figure 10–4.**  The plantar fascia.

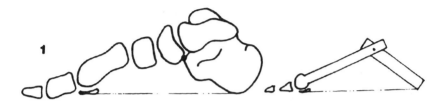

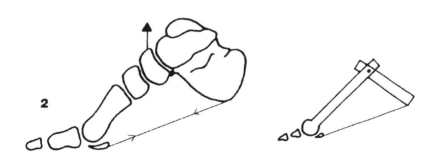

**Figure 10–5.** The windlass effect on the longitudinal arch of the foot:
(1) windlass effect, and (2) elevation of the longitudinal arch as a result
of the windlass effect (adapted from Basmajian, 1975).

- The pain is slow in onset.
- Pain is increased in weightbearing activities.
- The pain may extend along the medial longitudinal arch.
- The pain is often worse on getting up in the morning.
- There is tenderness on palpation at the insertion of the plantar fascia on the calcaneum and there may be other points of tenderness along its extent.
- A significant decrease in the active and passive range of motion of extension and of passive flexion, of the first metatarsophalangeal joint has been noted in runners with this condition (Creighton & Olson, 1987).

## Treatment Guidelines

As with all repetitive strain injuries a decrease in weightbearing activities and ice application are useful in the treatment of this condition. In addition the following treatments have proved beneficial:

- stretching and ultrasound;
- support in terms of the low dye strapping technique (Kosmahl & Kosmahl, 1987; Torg, 1990) until the acute pain has subsided;
- weight bearing with the strapping in place;
- heel pads;
- orthotics to correct the biomechanical problem.

## B. MEDIAL TARSAL TUNNEL SYNDROME (MTTS)

Medial tarsal tunnel syndrome was first reported by Kick (1962) and Lam (1962). It is a compression syndrome affecting the posterior tibial nerve or its branches. The compression occurs in the medial tarsal tunnel, which is a fibro-osseous tunnel situated just posterior to the medial malleolus. The roof of the tunnel is formed by a fan shaped sheet of fibrous tissue called the medial retinaculum.

## Etiology

Kushner and Reid (1984) identified a number of circumstances in which the condition might occur. These are listed under the headings of anatomical, trauma, tumor, and miscellaneous. This etiological classification was later reiterated by Reid (1990). Included in the classification are such causes as fractures, dislocations, and inflammatory conditions. Jackson and Haglund (1992) describe the condition as an overuse syndrome in runners, and feel that abnormal biomechanical factors, such as excessive pronation or valgus, could be the causative agents.

## Clinical Features

The clinical features will vary in accordance with the branch of the nerve that is being subjected to pressure. If the symptoms are on the medial side of the foot the medial plantar nerve is the culprit; symptoms on the lateral side of the foot would implicate the lateral plantar nerve. If pain in the heel is a major factor the medial calcaneal branch (a branch from the sural nerve) may have been subjected to pressure. The medial plantar nerve is the one which is most often affected. The following features may be present.

- There may be paresthesia and a burning pain on the plantar surface of the foot, commonly affecting the great toe.
- The patient may complain of a swollen or tight feeling.
- The pain is often worse at night causing the patient to walk around or to rub the foot to gain relief.
- When the posterior tibial nerve is tapped the symptoms increase (positive Tinel's sign).
- A diminished two point discrimination response may be present.
- In the chronic state weakness of the muscles supplied by the median plantar nerve may develop.

## Treatment Guidelines

The condition usually responds to a non-surgical approach.

- Ice and ultrasound are used to control the pain and reduce fibrosis.
- Correction of adverse training errors such as excessive mileage and inappropriate footwear is essential.
- An orthotic device may be used to correct biomechanical problems.

If the above approach fails, surgery will be performed, in the form of a decompression procedure such as incising the flexor retinaculum.

## C. FAT PAD SYNDROME

The heel pad is a structure composed of lobules of fat, which are accommodated in septal compartments beneath the heel. Its function is to absorb compression forces during weight bearing. With aging the fat lobules decrease and greater stress is placed on the fascial septa and the underlying bone, resulting in a painful response on weight bearing. This response is compounded if the heel is subjected to repetitive stress, as in running, or to additional pressure from biomechanical abnormalities.

### Treatment Guidelines

Rest, ice, heel pad support, and correction of training methods are useful approaches in the treatment of this condition.

The most common causes of pain beneath the heel have been identified and addressed. If pain persists following treatment, involvement of the medial calcaneal nerve to the heel should be suspected.

*Note:* Baxter, Pfeffer, and Thigpen (1989) report on the entrapment of the first branch of the lateral plantar nerve as a frequently overlooked cause of pain beneath the heel. The nerve supplies muscle, but it also has a sensory component to the periosteum of the medial calcaneal tuberosity; Baxter and his colleagues feel that entrapment of this nerve is responsible for 20 per cent of chronic heel pain.

### PAIN AT THE SIDES OF THE HEEL

Tenosynovitis is an inflammatory condition affecting the sheaths of tendons (Figure 10–3). At the sides of the heel the **sheath of tibialis posterior tendon** on the medial side, and the **sheath of the peronei** on the lateral side can become inflamed, giving rise to pain. These two conditions will be discussed independently.

### A. TIBIALIS POSTERIOR TENOSYNOVITIS

Tibialis posterior tenosynovitis is a fairly common disorder in runners, particularly in those with excessive pronation of the foot.

## Mechanism of Injury

This is a repetitive strain injury in the runner whose foot moves into excessive pronation, or who has a valgus deformity of the hind foot. It can develop in non-athletic people with the same biomechanical problems.

## Clinical Features

The problem usually develops below or behind the medial malleolus.

- There is tenderness on palpation over the tendon and swelling is evident.
- Resisted inversion of the foot and passive eversion will increase the pain.
- Crepitus may be felt.
- The patient complains of major discomfort in the weight-bearing position.

## B. PERONEAL TENOSYNOVITIS

Peroneal tenosynovitis may develop anywhere from behind the lateral malleolus to the insertion of the peroneus brevis tendon into the base of the fifth metatarsal.

## Mechanism of Injury

The condition develops as a result of irritation to the tendon sheath from excessive eversion and dorsiflexion.

## Clinical Features

The clinical features are similar to tibialis posterior tenosynovitis in terms of tenderness on palpation and crepitus, except that both will be experienced behind the lateral malleolus. Those features that are specific to peroneal tenosynovitis are:

- pain on stretching the tendon during passive inversion;
- pain on resisted eversion.

## Treatment Guidelines

Treatment guidelines are similar for both conditions and involve rest, ice, ultrasound, and correction of the irritating factor. In the case of tibialis posterior tenosynovitis caused by excessive pronation an orthotic device to correct the problem is often warranted.

## PAIN WITHIN THE HEEL

Adams and Hamblen (1990) suggest that pain within the heel is attributable either to arthritis of the subtalar joint or to pathology affecting the calcaneum. These sources of pain are mentioned so that the reader will take these two possibilities into account when differentiating between the different causes of pain in and around the heel.

## METATARSALGIA

The word metatarsalgia means pain in the region of the metatarsals. The most common cause of this pain is collapse of the transverse arch.

## A. COLLAPSE OF THE TRANSVERSE ARCH

Undue pressure on the transverse arch causes its collapse with resultant painful callosities on the second, third, and fourth metatatarsal heads. Conservative treatment involves soaking the feet and removing the accumulated dead skin forming the callosities. A metatarsal pad placed just proximal to the metatarsal heads will help to reduce further pressure, as will avoidance of high heeled shoes. Sometimes it is necessary to surgically implement a sling support to the arch.

## MORTON'S NEUROMA

Morton's neuroma is pressure on the digital nerve usually between the 3rd and 4th metatarsals. It was thought that the pressure was caused by a neuroma, but Welsh (1990) has suggested that the pressure may stem from an involvement of the bursa in the region. The condition produces pain on the adjacent sides of the toes supplied by the digital nerve that is being subjected to pressure. Treatment involves releasing the pressure by conservative means such as a metatarsal pad (Adams & Hamblen, 1990); otherwise surgical intervention is necessary to remove the offending neuroma or bursa.

## DEFORMITIES OF THE TOES

Toe deformities are fairly common, particularly those relating to the great toe. The latter have significance in terms of the normal weightbearing function of the great toe. It will be recalled that the plantar fascia functions as a windlass when the first metatarsophalangeal (MTP) joint goes into dorsiflexion at the heel off phase of gait. In so doing the proximal phalanx glides up over the MT head causing the first metatarsal to go into plantar flexion (Mann, 1989).

Problems involving the great toe are more common in women than in men and it is felt that inappropriate footwear is the major causative factor.

## A. HALLUX VALGUS

Hallux valgus is a condition in which the great toe is deviated laterally at the metatarsophalangeal joint and the first metatarsal deviates medially (Figure 10–6). Consequently there is a lateral subluxation of the joint and there is a greater space than is normal between the first and second metatarsal heads. A painful bursitis or exostosis develops on the medial aspect of the joint. The normal hallux valgus angle (that formed by the intersection of a line through the long axis of the metatarsal and one through the proximal phalanx) should be less than 15° (Mann, 1989). Hallux valgus is much more common in women than in men and is thought to be the result of inappropriate foot wear.

### Treatment

In the early stages of the condition protecting the exostosis from pressure, by using appropriate footwear (with an enlarged toe section) is helpful, but as the condition progresses surgery to correct the deformity is the only answer.

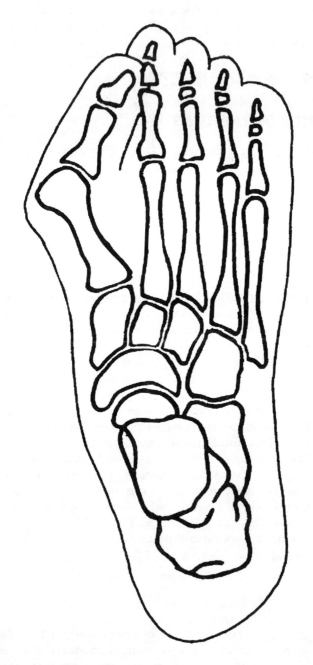

**Figure 10–6.**  Hallux valgus.

*Note:* Mann (1989) has pointed out that selection of a surgical procedure that does not interfere with the windlass mechanism of the foot is important.

## B. HALLUX RIGIDUS

In the condition known as hallux rigidus there is ankylosis of the first metatarsophalangeal joint. In the early stages of development, before ankylosis takes place (hallux limitus), there is painful subluxation, in a plantar direction, of the proximal phalanx on the first metatarsal. The ankylosis occurs in older people as a result of degenerative changes. On ankylosis of the joint the painful symptoms usually subside.

## SUMMARY

At the onset of this chapter an attempt was made to clarify some of the complex biomechanical aspects of the talocrural joint, the sub-talar joint and the mid-tarsal joint, their interrelationships with each other and with the lower extremity. Lateral Ligament Sprain was selected as the most common soft tissue affliction of the talocrural joint. Conditions responsible for pain in and around the heel were discussed next, starting with those causing posterior heel pain, for instance Achilles Tendinitis, followed by those causing inferior heel pain, such as Plantar Fasciitis. The Medial Tarsal Tunnel Syndrome and Tibialis Posterior Tenosynovitis presented problems for discussion on the medial aspect of the foot and heel, whereas Peroneal Tenosynovitis presented an inflammatory problem of tendons and their sheaths at the lateral side of the heel. The chapter ended with some common problems of the foot including Metatarsalgia and Hallux Valgus.

# CHAPTER 11

# Introduction to Fractures

This chapter is based upon the work of Adams (1968), Apley (1973), Huckstep (1978), and McRae, (1981).

## BASIC CONCEPTS

A fracture is present when there is a break in the continuity of the cortex of the bone. Next to soft tissue injuries, fractures are the most common injuries associated with the musculoskeletal system. Physical therapists do not treat fractures as such, but they are responsible for the rehabilitation of the patient when the fracture has united, or, less commonly, participate in the process of facilitating union of a fracture. The rehabilitation involves restoring the damaged soft tissue structures to their normal physiological and functional ability as well as promoting bone consolidation.

The terminology relating to fractures is complex and often confusing and so this chapter will begin with basis concepts, including a classification of the types of fractures and other definitions relating to their treatment. The second section deals with common fractures of the extremities.

## Classification of Fractures

Fractures are classified in terms of their complexity.

### Simple Fracture (Closed)

In simple closed fractures the skin remains intact and the fracture is not exposed to the exterior; the chances of infection are therefore decreased. The term **simple** bears no relation to the severity of the fracture.

### Compound Fracture (Open)

In open compound fractures there is a **break in the skin**, because of a sustained external wound; consequently the tissues are exposed to outside organisms and the chances of infection are greatly increased. The skin can be broken by the object producing the force, that is, from some external force, or by a bony fragment of the fracture penetrating the skin by protruding outward from the fracture site.

## Classification of Causes of Fractures

Essentially there are three different causes of fractures, namely trauma, bone pathology, and stress. The most common of these is trauma (i.e., violence).

### Trauma

Fractures sustained by violence can be subdivided into two groups.

**Direct Trauma.** With this mechanism the fracture is sustained at the point of contact of the violent force, for instance, a fracture of the shaft of the femur at the point of contact with a moving car.

**Indirect Trauma.** Here the fracture is sustained at a distance from the point of contact of the violent force, for example, a fracture of the clavicle from a fall on the outstretched hand.

### Bone Pathology

A pathological bone fracture is caused by disease of bone or by metastasis of a tumor. The presence of either weakens the bone making it susceptible to even slight stresses which result in a fracture. Osteoporosis of the hip or the thoracic spine often results in fractures in these regions.

### Stress

Stress is another cause of fractures. With stress fractures the bone is subjected to repetitive stresses that ultimately result in a fracture of the bone. An example of this type of fracture is the "march" fracture of the second metatarsal, associated with soldiers. The repetitive stresses from marching result in a stress fracture of the metatarsal. The fracture can be sustained at the point of the repetitive stress or at a distance from it. The type of fracture sustained is usually a hair-line fracture which can be difficult to detect even on an X-ray.

Fractures developing as a result of bone pathology or repetitive stress are not as common as those caused by trauma. Fractures developing from pathological causes such as metastasis, or osteoporosis of the thoracic spine, are difficult to treat whereas repetitive stress usually results in a fracture that is relatively easy to treat.

## Anatomical Location of the Fracture

The shaft of a long bone is arbitrarily divided into three parts. The fracture can then be described as lying in the upper, middle, or lower third of the shaft. It may also be described as lying at the level of the junction of the upper and middle thirds.

## Patterns of a Fracture

Fractures assume a variety of patterns (Figures 11–1 and 11–2) that may influence their stability and rate of healing.

### Greenstick

Greensticks are a type of fracture occurring in children, usually from indirect trauma, such as a longitudinal compression force in which the bone crumples on one side, or an angulation force where the bone may bend on one side and crack on the other.

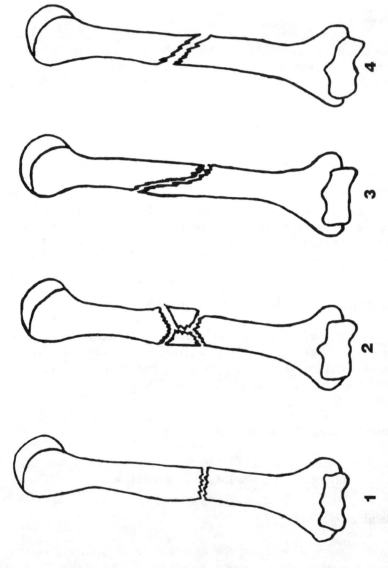

**Figure 11–1.** Patterns of simple fractures of the humerus: (1) transverse, (2) comminuted, (3) spiral, and 4) oblique.

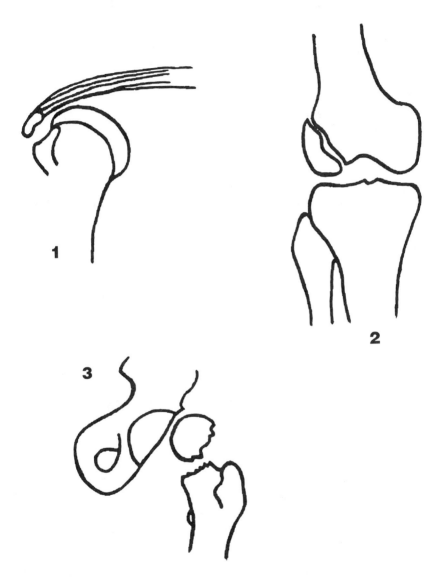

**Figure 11–2.** Patterns of complex fractures: (1) avulsion fracture of the greater tuberosity of the humerus, (2) intra-articular fracture of the lateral condyle of the femur, and (3) fracture dislocation of the neck of the femur (adapted from McRae, 1981).

### Transverse

Transverse fractures are usually caused by direct trauma, but may also be caused by an indirect angular force. The fracture extends from one side of the bone to the other.

### Oblique

Oblique fractures are usually caused by indirect trauma. The fracture line lies oblique to the bone axis.

### Spiral

Spiral fractures are caused by indirect trauma; the bone is twisted on its long axis.

### Comminuted

Comminuted fractures present with more than two fragments; they are caused by either direct or indirect trauma.

### Impacted

Indirect trauma is usually the cause of impacted fractures. The fragments are driven into each other and remain locked together.

### Crush

In crush fractures the causative factor is direct or indirect trauma; it always involves cancellous bone which has only a thin cortical cover. An example of this type of fracture would be a crush fracture of the calcaneum as a result of landing on the heels when falling from a height.

### Avulsion

Excessive stress applied to a tendon or ligament can produce an injury, called an avulsion fracture, in which the soft tissue structure and a fragment of bone are pulled from the parent bone.

### Fracture into the Joint

Fracture into the joint occurs when the fracture involves the articular surface of the joint; from the viewpoint of rehabilitation and joint complications it is one of the most difficult to treat.

### Fracture-Dislocation

A fracture-dislocation is accompanied by dislocation of the joint.

## Stability of Fractures

Fractures may be either stable or unstable. In the stable fracture there is either no displacement, or no danger of re-displacement following reduction. Stability depends upon three factors:

1. the direction of the line of the fracture;
2. the forces applied by muscle pull;
3. the integrity of ligaments.

### 1. The Line of the Fracture

The following fractures are considered stable:

- transverse fractures with bayonet apposition in which a spike of bone from one fragment is inserted into the other creating a partial impaction;
- greenstick fractures;
- impacted fractures.

The following fractures are considered unstable:

- spiral fractures with a slope of more than 20°;
- oblique fractures;
- comminuted fractures (unless impacted).

### 2. Muscle Pull

When the muscle pull is unbalanced redisplacement may occur; for example, oblique fractures of the humerus below the insertion of deltoid are unstable because of the unbalanced action of this muscle.

### 3. Integrity of Ligaments

Stability of the joints depends on the integrity of the ligaments; therefore, fracture-dislocations with inevitable tearing of the ligaments are unstable.

## Resulting Displacements

A variety of displacements can develop as a result of a fracture (Figure 11–3); these are described in relation to the displacement of the bony fragments, producing an abnormal anatomical alignment. The deformity is described in terms of the shift of the distal fragment, but is determined by the following factors:

- the nature of the violence causing the fracture;
- the direction in which it is applied;
- the subsequent effects of gravity and muscle pull.

### Angulation

Angulation occurs when the bony fragments form an angle to each other. The angulation is described in terms of the position of the point of the angle; for instance, if the point of the angle is directed posteriorly the fracture would be described as a posterior angulation.

### Rotation

In rotation fractures the distal fragment is rotated, usually in its long axis.

### Partial Displacement

In partial displacement the distal fragment (usually of a transverse fracture) shifts from its axial alignment because of transverse rotation or angulation, but there is still some contact between the bone ends.

### Overlap or Shortening

In overlap (shortening) fractures there is complete displacement enabling fragments to overlap, with resultant shortening.

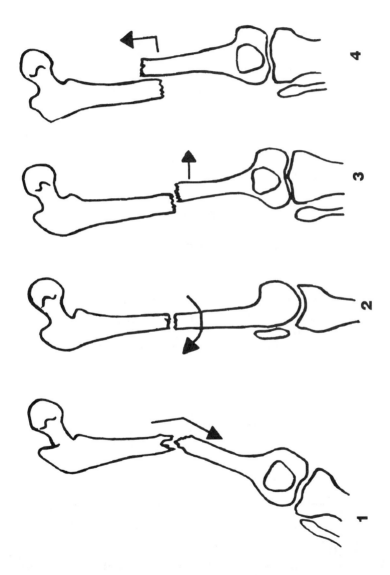

**Figure 11–3.** Fracture displacements of the femur: (1) angulation, (2) rotation, (3) medial displacement, and (4) over-riding (adapted from McRae, 1981).

*Bayonet Apposition*

In bayonet apposition a spike of bone from one fragment penetrates the medullary cavity of the other. Lateral displacement is present, but the fracture is stable.

## Associated Injuries

Inevitably with fractures there will be associated physiological reactions to damage and a varied symptomatology; these are described below.

### Shock

Shock is a component part of most severe injuries. It can be divided into primary and secondary shock.

**Primary Shock.**   This may occur immediately; vaso-constricting nerves are inhibited, and peripheral vessels dilate. There is insufficient blood to fill them, the blood pressure drops, and the patient becomes pale and faints. Spontaneous recovery occurs in a few minutes.

**Secondary Shock.**   This condition develops later and is usually brought on by hemorrhage. It is a fairly common occurrence after fractures of long bones because medullary blood vessels are torn and there is free bleeding into the tissues. The reduction of blood volume is compensated for by contraction of peripheral blood vessels. The skin becomes pale, cold, and moist and the heart beats faster; recovery is prompt if the blood volume is restored by transfusion. The blood required is two pints for each fractured femur plus one for each fractured tibia, humerus, and forearm bone.

### Ischemia

Ischemia may follow injury of a main artery and it is important to check the signs and symptoms listed below.

- The pulse may be weak or absent.
- During the next 4 hours it is important to check temperature — "a very cold" feeling of fingers or toes, and the "4p's": paresthesia (or numbness), pallor, pain, and paralysis.

*Note:* See Volkmann's Ischemic Contracture later in this chapter.

### Visceral Injuries

The most common visceral injuries are those related to the bladder, the spleen, and the pleurae.

### Joints

Associated with the fracture there may be a dislocation of the joints: this needs to be determined as soon as possible.

### Nerve Injuries

Nerve injuries may be associated with fractures and it is important to check the skin sensation and any extreme loss of muscle power.

### Muscles

Muscles may be injured in terms of strain or partial or complete rupture.

## Clinical Features

The clinical features of a fracture are fairly consistent; they are listed below:

- tenderness over the bone;
- swelling;
- deformity—visible or palpable;
- loss of function;
- visible bruising.

## Principles of Treatment

The first principle of treatment of the fracture is to deal with any associated life-threatening situation such as shock or hemorrhage. Following this the displaced fracture is reduced, then immobilized.

## Reduction

The second principle is the restoration of the bony fragments to normal alignment. The procedure is unnecessary when there is no displacement. Reduction is achieved either by closed reduction or by open reduction. Closed reduction will be discussed first.

**Closed Reduction.** This is achieved by manual manipulation under general anesthetic. It is called closed reduction because there is no surgical intervention and it is the preferred method for these reasons:

- no further damage is inflicted on soft tissues by surgical intervention;
- there is no risk of infection;
- the hematoma is undisturbed.

The **procedure** for achieving a successful closed reduction with the patient under anesthetic is as follows:

- study of the displacement on X-ray;
- application of traction in a longitudinal direction;
- separation of the fragments in impacted fractures;
- application of corrective forces;
- restoration of normal alignment, as much as is possible.

**Open Reduction.** This procedure involves surgical intervention and is used under the following circumstances:

- internal fixation with screws, wires, rods, and other mechanical means is required because the fracture cannot be held together by any other method (Figure 11–4);
- perfect apposition of the bony fragments is desirable, for instance where the fracture involves the articular surface of a joint;
- open reduction is used where closed reduction has failed;
- open reduction may also be preferred in order to avoid long periods of bed rest, as for example in an elderly patient.

## Immobilization

Immobilization is the third principle of fracture treatment. It involves immobilizing the reduced fracture fragments, for instance

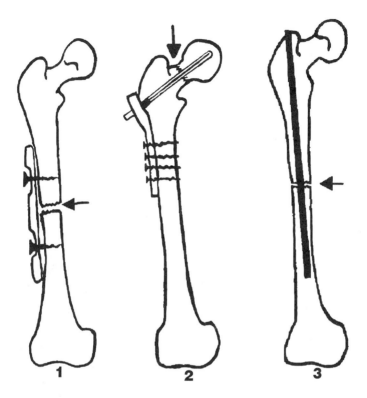

**Figure 11–4.** Methods of internal fixation: (1) plate and screws for a transverse fracture of the femoral shaft; (2) nail, plate, and screws for a fracture of the neck of femur; and (3) intramedullary rod for a fracture of the shaft of femur (adapted from McRae, 1981).

by placing the fractured limb in a cast. The purpose of immobilization is to maintain the position of the fracture fragments and to prevent movement across the fracture site. The joint above the fracture and the joint below are usually immobilized. It is not necessary for all fractures, but is essential for most fractures of long bones and for unstable fractures.

It was mentioned previously that one way to immobilize a fracture was by means of a plaster cast, which is the most common method used. Other methods (Figure 11–5) include:

- slings; these are commonly used for upper extremity fractures;
- walking casts and cast bracing which are used for lower extremity fractures;

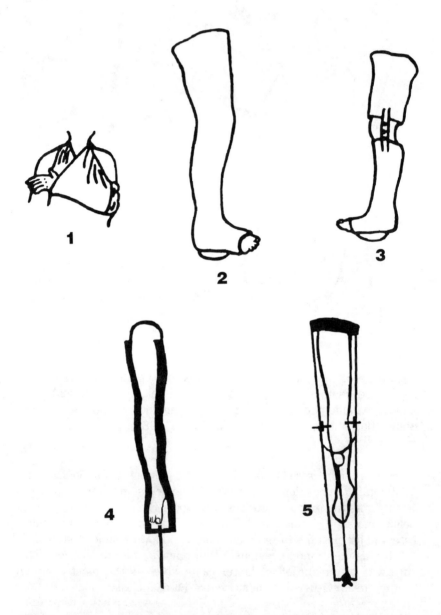

**Figure 11–5.** Methods of immobilization: (1) sling, (2) above knee walking plaster, (3) hinge walking plaster, (4) skin traction, and (5) skeletal traction (adapted from Huckstep, 1978 and McRae, 1981).

- traction, applied by means of the skin (useful for children's fractures);
- skeletal traction, where the traction is applied by means of a pin (for instance, the Steinman pin) inserted into bone. The traction force is transmitted through a series of ropes and pulleys. This method is used in fractures of the shaft of the femur.

### Effects of Exercise

It was stated earlier that the physical therapist is not usually involved in the treatment of the unreduced fracture; however, during the immobilization phase, he or she is very much involved in the rehabilitation process, including soft tissue mobilization. One of the methods of treatment is the implementation of exercises that the patient must perform regularly. The effects of exercise are as follows:

- promotion of edema absorption;
- prevention of organization of blood clots following hemorrhage;
- prevention of loss of elasticity of muscles and thus of restriction of movement attributable to tightness in the antagonistic muscle group;
- prevention of formation of unnecessary scar tissue within a damaged muscle;
- maintenance of movement of joints not encased in plaster;
- maintenance of strength of muscles encased in plaster by the performance of isometric contractions;
- maintenance of an adequate circulation.

## Healing of Fractures

Once the fracture has been reduced and immobilized, if necessary, it heals in five stages (Figure 11–6).

### Clinical Union

Clinical union is the earliest stage of the process of union. It is present when there is a shadow on the X-ray and an **absence of movement across the fracture site** when the physician attempts passive movement and the **patient does not experience pain** (Salter, 1983). Clinical union corresponds to the third stage of fracture healing.

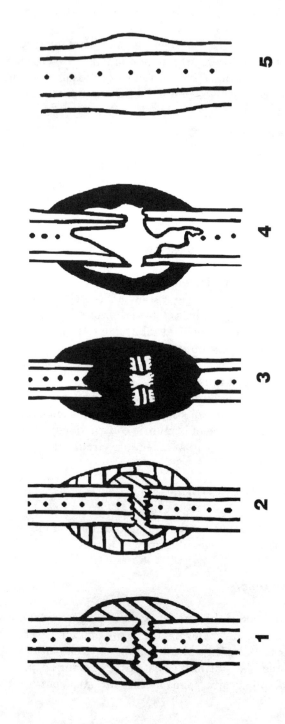

**Figure 11–6.** Stages of fracture healing: (1) hematoma formation, (2) cell proliferation, (3) woven bone, (4) lamellar bone, and (5) remodelling (adapted from Adams, 1968).

## Complications Associated with Fractures

Several complications can arise as a result of a fracture and many of these present problems for the physical therapist during the process of the patient's rehabilitation. Some of these complications are discussed below.

### Joint Stiffness

Joint stiffness is a very common complication following immobilization of the fracture. The problem relates to adhesion formation in the different tissues. These problems are:

- periarticular adhesions form as a result of deposition of fibrin in the surrounding tissue; it becomes fibrous tissue if left;
- intra-articular adhesions develop as a result of fibrin deposits between joint surfaces, or between these and capsules, or in synovial membrane, binding it together;
- muscular adhesions occur when there has been extensive soft tissue damage. Muscle and bone may be involved in the same hematoma and when this becomes organized they are tied firmly together by fibrous tissue.

### Injuries to Arteries and Nerves

Arteries and nerves can become injured by a fragment of the fracture or at the time the fracture was sustained.

### Problems with Union

Sometimes a fracture is slow in uniting; this is called delayed union, or it may unite by fibrous tissue; this is called non-union.

### Avascular Necrosis

Avascular necrosis results in death of bone because of interference with the blood supply, for example in the head of femur.

### Osteoarthritis

The condition of osteoarthritis is a fairly common complication of fractures involving joint surfaces.

# COMMON FRACTURES OF THE EXTREMITIES

In the following pages examples of common fractures of the upper and lower extremities are briefly described. It is not the author's intention to describe every common fracture of the extremities but rather to give the reader some insight into the mechanism of injury, the means of immobilization, and the complications that are specific to selected fractures.

# THE UPPER EXTREMITY

The upper extremity is a vulnerable part of the skeletal system where fractures are concerned. The cause is often indirect violence resulting from a fall on the outstretched hand.

## HUMERUS

Injuries to the humerus occur fairly frequently and will be described in terms of their location on the humerus (Figure 11–7).

## A. GREATER TUBEROSITY

In injuries to the greater tuberosity the type of fracture sustained is often comminuted.

### Mechanism of Injury

The mechanism of injury is usually direct violence, for example a fall or a blow to the shoulder.

### Method of Immobilization

Since this fracture is rarely displaced a collar and cuff or sling should be worn for 1–2 weeks until the acute symptoms have subsided, following which mobilization may commence.

## B. SURGICAL NECK

A surgical neck fracture is very common in the elderly.

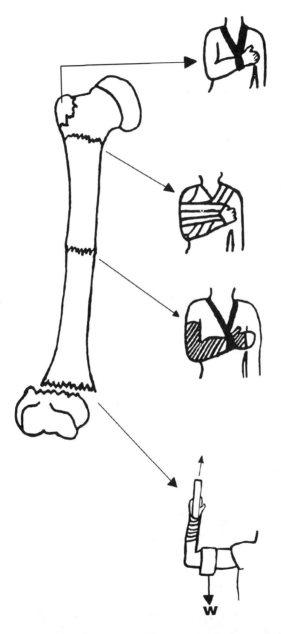

**Figure 11-7.** Fractures of the humerus and their methods of immobilization (adapted from Huckstep, 1978 and McRae, 1981).

## Mechanism of Injury

This fracture is sustained from indirect violence such as a fall on the outstretched hand.

## Method of Immobilization

Surgical neck fracture is usually impacted and is immobilized in a sling until the acute pain subsides. Exercises are commenced as soon as possible because of the danger of adhesive capsulitis. Non-impacted fractures require a more extensive and prolonged method of immobilization, such as having the arm bandaged across the trunk.

## C. SHAFT

A shaft type of fracture is usually displaced by the pull of associated muscles.

It can occur in the upper one third of the shaft, the middle of the shaft, or the lower one third of the shaft.

## Mechanism of Injury

This type of injury is sustained by indirect or direct violence.

## Method of Immobilization

A U slab of plaster is used that embraces the patient's flexed elbow and upper arm and extends to the point of the shoulder. The arm is then enclosed in a sling beneath the patient's clothes for about 6 weeks.

*Note:* It is important to watch for signs of radial nerve involvement, particularly with a mid-shaft fracture.

## D. SUPRACONDYLAR

Fractures of the supracondylar region are a common fracture in children up to the age of 8 years but they are seldom seen in adults. The upper fragment of the fracture may cause occlusion of the brachial artery with disastrous results. It is imperative that the hand be monitored for recognition of circulatory interference. If a cast has been applied it must be removed as soon as the signs of brachial artery occlusion are detected; traction is then applied (Figure 11–7). The blood supply to the flexors of the forearm and the nerves can be cut off causing a **Volkmann's ischemic contracture** (Figure 4–3).

## Mechanism of Injury

The cause is usually a fall on the outstretched hand.

## Method of Immobilization

If the fracture is undisplaced, a simple cast extending from below the axilla to the metacarpophalangeal (MCP) joints, with the elbow in approximately 90° of flexion, is applied and retained for three weeks. While in the cast the patient can perform exercises for the shoulder and fingers. Following immobilization exercises may be commenced for the joints that were enclosed in the cast.

Complicated fractures of the supracondylar region (Figure 11–7) might initially warrant traction immobilization (Huckstep, 1978; McRae, 1981).

## RADIUS AND ULNA

## A. SHAFTS

The shafts of the radius or ulna may be fractured independently, or both bones may sustain a fracture simultaneously.

## Mechanism of Injury

The fracture is caused by a fall on the outstretched hand (indirect violence) or by a direct blow.

## Method of Immobilization

If both bones have been broken an accurate reduction is necessary to retain the integrity of the interrelated movement of the radius and ulna. The limb is then placed in a full length cast with the elbow at 90° flexion and the forearm mid-way between pronation and supination, for a period of 8 to 12 weeks.

If a closed reduction is not obtainable an open reduction is attempted and the fragments are maintained by internal fixation, for example plates, screws, or intramedullary pins. A cast may be applied for 6 weeks.

## B. COLLES FRACTURE

Colles fracture is an extremely common fracture of the lower end of the radius (Figure 11–8) in the 40 years-plus age group. It occurs about 2 cm above the wrist. The fracture is commonly displaced in a typical fashion in that the distal fragment is displaced dorsally and laterally with a backward tilt. This deformity is commonly called the "dinner fork deformity." Less commonly there is a crack fracture without displacement. In severe comminuted fractures external and internal fixation with screws and pins may be required.

## Mechanism of Injury

Once again the cause of injury is indirect trauma; the fracture is sustained by a fall on the outstretched hand.

## Method of Immobilization

In severe fractures the plaster cast may extend from above the elbow to just proximal to the MCP joints. The wrist is in slight flexion and ulnar deviation to accommodate the swelling and to maintain the reduction. The cast is worn for approximately 6 weeks but may be changed to a cast below the elbow with the wrist in neutral position prior to the termination of the immobilization period.

If a crack fracture only has been sustained, the initial cast extends from below the elbow with the wrist in neutral position or slight extension, and is worn for about 4 weeks.

*Note:* There are some complications associated with this type of fracture that are worthy of consideration.

**Sudek's atrophy** (reflex sympathetic dystrophy) occasionally develops in the wrist and hand following removal of the cast. The signs and symptoms of reflex sympathetic dystrophy have been discussed previously in Chapter 4.

**Rupture of the extensor pollicis longus tendon** has been known to occur because of friction over the site of the fracture.

**Stiffness of shoulder and fingers** will develop if the patient is not instructed to use them while the limb is in the cast; this complication is common, as the patient is often elderly.

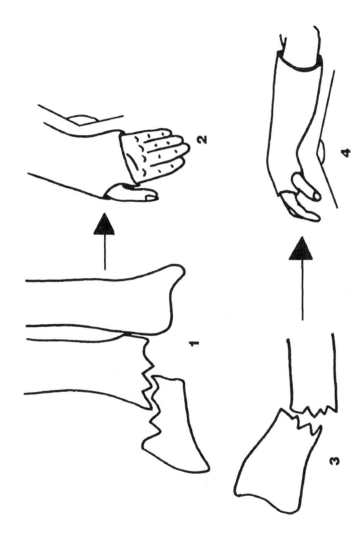

**Figure 11–8.** Colles' fracture and immobilization: (1) radial shift of distal fragment, (2) immobilization in ulnar deviation, (3) dorsal shift of the distal fragment, and (4) immobilization in wrist flexion (adapted from McRae, 1981).

## CARPUS

The most common fracture of the carpals is a fracture of the scaphoid bone.

## A. SCAPHOID

Scaphoid fracture is a fairly common fracture in the young adult and occurs most often across the middle of the bone or the waist. Fractures occurring here are prone to avascular necrosis because of interference in the blood supply at the fracture site. Often fractures of the scaphoid are hair-line and difficult to detect on X-ray and as a result they can be missed.

### Mechanism of Injury

A fall on the outstretched hand is a common mechanism of injury.

### Method of Immobilization

The fracture is immobilized by the application of a plaster cast extending from just below the elbow to below the metacarpophalangeal joints of the fingers, but extending to just below the interphalangeal joint of the thumb. The cast is maintained for 2 to 3 months, but is removed for reassessment and re-applied during this period.

*Note:* As mentioned previously avascular necrosis may be a complication of this type of fracture. In addition Sudek's atrophy and non-union or delayed union may exist.

## METACARPUS AND PHALANGES

Injuries of the metacarpals and phalanges cause swelling and it is imperative that this be controlled as soon as possible after the injury. It is often necessary for the patient to be admitted to the hospital if there are multiple fractures or extensive soft tissue damage. The patient's hand may be elevated, utilizing a roll towel or stockinette attached to an intravenous drip stand. The swelling must not be allowed to develop into chronic edema and resulting fibrosis.

Minor swelling can be controlled with an arm sling applied in such a way that the hand is positioned across the chest and well above the elbow. Exercises to the shoulder, elbow, and free fingers may be performed two to three times a day.

## A. BENNETT'S FRACTURE-DISLOCATION

Bennett's fracture-dislocation occurs at the first metacarpal on the trapezium. The base of the thumb sustains the fracture, resulting in a small medial fragment that remains in contact with the trapezium, and a large lateral fragment that dislocates.

### Mechanism of Injury

The fracture is caused either by a fall, or by a blow on the clenched fist, or by a forced abduction of the thumb.

### Method of Immobilization

The thumb is held in the abducted position and traction is applied. The cast extends from just below the elbow to proximal to the metacarpophalangeal joints of the fingers and just proximal to the interphalangeal joint of the thumb. It is maintained for approximately 6 weeks. Open reduction and internal fixation may be the chosen method of immobilization.

*Note*: Fractures of the metacarpals and phalanges of the fingers are treated with minimum immobilization to the unaffected part of the hand. This is to ensure that the function of the hand is maintained as much as possible while the injured part is adequately protected.

## THE LOWER EXTREMITY

Fractures of the long bones of the lower extremity are often the result of extreme violence such as a motor vehicle accident (MVA). Some of the most common fractures relate to the femur and these will be discussed first.

# FEMUR

Fractures of the neck and shaft of the femur (Figure 11–9) will be described next.

## A. NECK

Neck fractures are very common in the elderly because of the presence of osteoporosis. There are four different types, two are intracapsular and two are extracapsular. The intracapsular fractures are the **subcapital**, which occurs at the most proximal part of the neck of the femur, and the **transcervical**, which occurs across the middle of the neck of the femur.

Extracapsular fractures are those which are either located at the base of the neck or those which involve one or both of the trochanters.

## Mechanism of Injury

These fractures are caused most often by a rotational force when the patient slips and falls.

## Method of Immobilization

Initially the patient will be on traction to prevent further displacement of the fragments and to allow some time to bring the patient to the optimum state for surgery. Analgesics and other medications may be administered. The fracture is treated by internal fixation in order to minimize bed rest and to mobilize the patient as quickly as possible. Depending upon the type of fracture the surgeon may elect to utilize a trifin nail, a compression screw, pins, pin and plate, femoral arthroplasty, or a total hip replacement. Early weightbearing is encouraged.

## B. SHAFT

A shaft fracture can occur in any part of the shaft.

## Mechanism of Injury

The injury is usually caused by direct trauma and the fracture may be simple or compound.

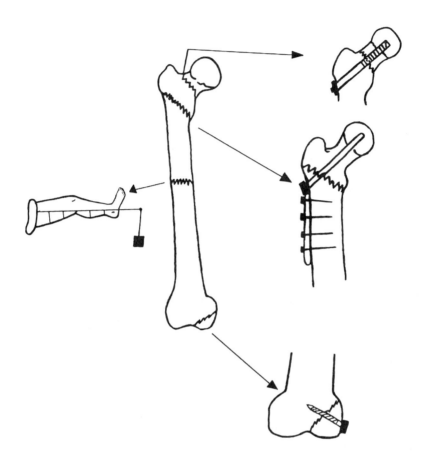

**Figure 11–9.** Fractures of the femur and their methods of immobilization (adapted from Huckstep, 1978 and McRae, 1981).

## Method of Immobilization

A Thomas splint is used initially with skeletal traction, after which a cast brace may be applied, with the hinges locked, for early weightbearing. After 1 or 2 weeks knee movement can begin and the crutches are gradually discarded. Alternatively internal fixation with an intramedullary rod may be selected instead of the Thomas splint. Internal fixation is almost essential in fractures involving the upper one third because of the pull of psoas and the glutei on the proximal fragment. Open reduction with internal fixation could be the chosen method of immobilization.

## PATELLA

Patellar fractures can be transverse, longitudinal, or of a crush type.

## Mechanism of Injury

The mechanism of injury can be either direct trauma, for example when the flexed knee strikes the dashboard in a MVA resulting in a crush fracture, or indirect trauma such as a strong muscle pull of the quadriceps. The latter can cause a transverse fracture of the patella.

## Method of Immobilization

A plaster cylinder is usually applied with the knee in extension for a period of 6 weeks.

## TIBIA AND FIBULA

Fractures of the tibia and fibula are not uncommon (Figure 11–10). They may be fractured independently or simultaneously. A fracture of the tibia can pose a major problem in terms of union and a fracture of the fibula can be relatively straightforward, although it too can create problems in terms of union.

## A. TIBIAL PLATEAU

A tibial plateau type of fracture occurs as a result of the femoral condyle coming into violent contact with the corresponding tibial plateau.

## Mechanism of Injury

The causative mechanism is either a valgus force producing a lateral tibial plateau fracture or a varus force resulting in a medial tibial plateau fracture.

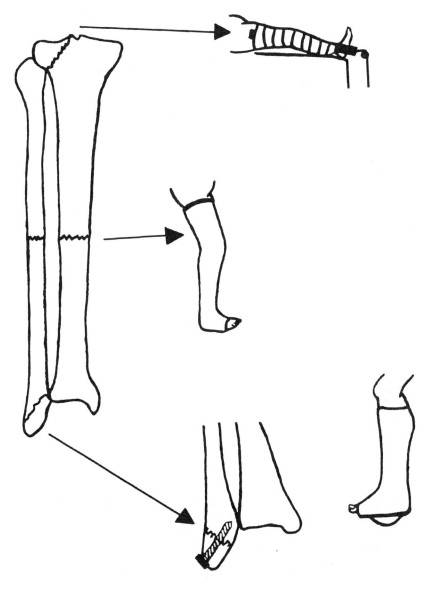

**Figure 11–10.** Fractures of the tibia and fibula and their methods of immobilization (adapted from McRae, 1981).

## Method of Immobilization

If the fracture is not complicated by damage to the soft tissue structures, skin traction is applied for about 4 weeks. During this time the patient is encouraged to perform quadriceps exercises as soon as possible, and knee flexion exercises when the pain subsides. Following the period on skin traction the patient is non-weight-bearing for a further 4 weeks. Open reduction with internal fixation may be the surgeon's choice for immobilization.

## B. SHAFTS OF THE TIBIA AND FIBULA

As a general rule it is the fracture of the tibia that is treated first since this bone has major weightbearing functions. However, the fracture of the fibula must be reduced to act as a brace for the tibia.

## Mechanism of Injury

The causative mechanism can be either direct violence such as a MVA, or indirect violence such as torsional stress sustained during a sporting activity.

## Method of Immobilization

If the fractures are undisplaced, or only minimally displaced, a full length cast is applied with the knee in slight flexion. The limb is usually elevated to control swelling for 48 hours or so. The patient is allowed to leave the hospital when able to use crutches. A walking heel is incorporated into the cast when the fracture is stable, usually between 4 to 6 weeks, or a patellar weightbearing cast with the introduction of a rocker sole may be applied. It takes an average of 16 weeks for a tibial fracture to unite.

More complicated tibial fractures are dealt with either by internal or external fixation devices.

## C. MALLEOLI

A fractured malleolus is a common occurrence. It is much more common for the lateral malleolus to be fractured than the medial malleolus.

## Mechanism of Injury

The lateral malleolus can be avulsed by an adduction force or sheared off by a lateral rotation or abduction force.

The medial malleolus may be sheared off by an adduction force or avulsed by an abduction force.

## Method of Immobilization

In the case of the lateral malleolus, immobilization in a below knee walking cast for 3 to 6 weeks is all that is required. **Stable** fractures of the medial malleolus may be treated in a similar fashion. However, **unstable** fractures of either of the malleoli may involve open reduction with a screw fixation. The limb is immobilized in a below knee cast. The patient is usually retained in hospital for a few days to ensure that the swelling is controlled, then non-weight-bearing movement on crutches can commence. A walking heel can be incorporated at 6 weeks. Union takes 8 to 9 weeks.

# GENERAL PRINCIPLES OF REHABILITATION OF FRACTURES FOLLOWING IMMOBILIZATION

Quite often the post-immobilization stage is one of the most distressing for the patient in terms of pain, swelling, stiffness and muscle weakness. Yet this crucial stage in the outpatient management of fractures is often mishandled. The patient may not be referred to a physical therapist once the cast is removed; instead he or she is given vague instructions relating to "keeping the joints moving" by an intern or other member of the outpatient team. The result is that when they return to the outpatient department for a checkup they may do so with established joint stiffness, edema, and discoloration caused by circulatory problems and, if the fracture is in the lower extremity, an antalgic gait pattern. These signs and symptoms might have been avoided had the patient been referred to a physical therapist for careful instruction and demonstration of the required treatment program as soon as the cast was removed, with follow-up sessions for progression of the program.

## Swelling

The patient must be informed of the dangers of having the limb in the dependent position in terms of its effect on the circulatory system, manifested by increased distal swelling of the extremities. This is particularly so of fractures of the forearm and wrist, and of the leg and ankle. Elevation of the affected limb combined with a carefully taught exercise program performed several times each day will not only counteract the effects of dependency but will drastically reduce swelling and help to restore the normal physiology of the joint. The application of a tensor bandage in the non-dependent position will help to ensure that swelling is further controlled.

## Range of Motion and Strengthening Program

Exercises are not only directed at the affected part of the limb but must also include the joints above and below the fracture level, since they too may have been immobilized in order to maintain a good reduction of the fracture. Even if they have not been immobilized a proximal to distal approach to ensuring normal range of motion and strength is advisable. The joints of the limbs are interrelated and work in concert with each other; a proximal weakness or restriction of range will have a negative effect distally. There are many mobilizing and strengthening techniques that can be applied locally to joints and muscles. However, proprioceptive neuromuscular facilitation (PNF) is an excellent approach to use to gain range, strength, and coordination.

## Restoration of Function

Restoration of function is the long-term goal in any form of rehabilitation and throughout the program. As range and strength are restored they must be applied to functional activities. Patients with fractures of the lower extremity will need instruction in the restoration of a normal gait pattern; those with fractures of the upper extemity need sufficient range and strength so that the hand can be used effectively in space.

## SUMMARY

This chapter began with a classification of fractures, their causes, and the patterns created. This was followed by a description of the features that contribute to the stability of a fracture. Next there was a review of associated injuries, presentation of the clinical features of fractures, and discussion of principles of treatment. The stages of fracture healing and clinical union were introduced and comments were made about the complications associated with fractures. The remainder of the chapter was devoted to some common fractures of the upper and lower extremity, mechanism of injury, method of immobilization, and complications.

# References

Adams, J. C. (1968) *Outline of fractures* (5th ed). Edinburgh and London: E. & S. Livingstone Ltd.

Adams, J. C., & Hamblen, D. L. (1990). *Outline of orthopaedics* (11th ed.). Edinburgh: Churchill Livingstone.

Adams, M. A., & Hutton, W. C. (1980). The effect of posture on the role of the apophyseal joints in resisting intervertebral compressive forces. *Journal of Bone and Joint Surgery*, 62B, 358–362.

Aisenbrey, J. A. (1987). Exercise in the prevention and management of osteoporosis. *Physical Therapy*, 67:17, 1100–1104.

Amendola, R., & Rorabeck, C. H. (1990). Chronic exertional compartmental syndrome. In J. S. Torg, R. P. Welsh, & R. J. Shephard (Eds.), *Current therapy in sports medicine-2* (pp. 250-253). Toronto, Philadelphia: B. C. Decker Inc.

Anderson, J. A .D. (1987). Back pain and occupation. In M. I. Jayson (Ed.), *The lumbar spine and back pain* (3rd ed.), (pp. 16–36). Edinburgh: Churchill Livingstone.

Andrews, J. R., & Wilson, F. (1985). Valgus extension overload in the pitching elbow. In B. Zarins, J. R. Andrews, & W.G. Carson (Eds), *Injuries to the throwing arm* (pp. 250–257). Philadelphia: W. B. Saunders Company.

Apley, A. G. (1973). *A system of orthopaedics and fractures* (4th ed.). London: Butterworths.

Arnoldi, C. C., Brodsky, A. E., Cauchoix, J., Crock, H. V., Dommisse, G. F., Edgar, M. A., Gargano, F. P., Jacobson, R. E., Kirkaldy-Willis, W. H., Kurihara, A., Langenskiöld, A., Macnab, I., McIvor, G.W.D., Newman, P. H., Paine, K. W. E., Russin, L. A., sheldon, J., Tile, M., Urist, M. R., Wilson, W. E., & Wiltse, L. L. (1976). Lumbar stenosis and nerve root entrapment syndromes. *Clinical Orthopaedics and Related Research*, 115, 4–5.

Baslund, B., Thomsen, B. S., & Jensen, E. M. (1990). Frozen shoulder: Current concepts. *Scandinavian Journal of Rheumatology*, 19, 321–325.

Basmajian, J. V. (1975). *Grant's method of anatomy* (9th ed.). Baltimore: The Williams and Wilkins Company.

Bateman, J. E. (1972). *The shoulder and neck*. Philadelphia: W. B. Saunders.

Baugher, W. H., & White, G. M. (1985). Primary evaluation and management of knee injuries. *The Orthopedic Clinics of North America, 16:2*, 315–327.

Baxter, D. E., Pfeffer, G. B., & Thigpen, M. (1989). Chronic heel pain. Treatment rationale. *The Orthopedic Clinics of North America, 20:4*, 563–569.

Blackburn, T. A. (1985). The off-season program for the throwing arm. In B. Zarins, J. R. Andrews, & W. G. Carson (Eds.), *Injuries to the throwing arm* (pp. 277–292). Philadelphia: W. B. Saunders Company.

Bland, J. H. (1987). *Disorders of the cervical spine. Diagnosis and medical management*. Philadelphia: W.B. Saunders.

Blount, W. P., & Moe, J. H. (1980). *The Milwaukee brace* (2nd ed.). Baltimore: Williams and Wilkins.

Bogduk, N. (1986). The anatomy and physiology of whiplash. Review paper. *Clinical Biomechanics, 1*, 92–101.

Bogduk, N., & Twomey, L. T. (1991). *Clinical anatomy of the lumbar spine* (2nd ed.). Edinburgh: Churchill Livingstone.

Brody, D. M. (1980). Running injuries. *Clinical Symposia, 32:4*. Summit, NJ.: CIBA Pharmaceutical Company.

Broom, M. J., & Fulkerson, J. P. (1986). The plica syndrome. A new perspective. *The Orthopedic Clinics of North America, 17:2*, 279-282.

Brown, D. E. (1990). Patellar dislocation, subluxation and the Elmslie-Trillat procedure. In J. S. Torg, R. P. Welsh, & R. J. Shephard (Eds.), *Current therapy in sports medicine-2* (pp. 275-277). Toronto, Philadelphia: B. C. Decker Inc.

Brownstein, B., Mangine, R. W., Noyes, F. R., & Kryger, S. (1988). Anatomy and biomechanics. In R.E. Mangine (Ed.), *Clinics in physical therapy. Volume 19. Physical therapy of the knee* (pp. 1–30). New York: Churchill Livingstone.

Cailliet, R. (1966). *Shoulder pain*. Philadelphia: F. A. Davis Company.

Cailliet, R. (1988). *Soft tissue pain and disability* (2nd ed.). Philadelphia: F.A. Davis Company.

Carroll, R. E., & Hurst, L. C. (1982). The relationship of thoracic outlet syndrome and carpal tunnel syndrome. *Clinical Orthopaedics and Related Research, 164*, 149–153.

Carson, W. G. (1985). Extra-articular reconstruction of the anterior cruciate ligament: *Lateral procedures. The Orthopedic Clinics of North America, 16:2*, 191–211.

Chen, S. C. (1990). Patellar pain syndrome: Instability and lateral retinacular release. In J. S. Torg, R. P. Welsh, & R.J. Shephard (Eds.), *Current therapy in sports medicine-2* (pp. 267–271). Toronto and Philadelphia: B. C. Decker Inc.

Clancy, W. G., Jr. (1985a). Evaluation of acute knee injuries in athletes. *American Academy of Orthopaedic Surgeons. Symposium on Sports Medicine. The knee*. 185–193.

Clancy, W. G., Jr. (1985b). Conservative treatment of acute ligamentous injuries. *American Academy of Orthopaedic Surgeons. Symposium of Sports Medicine. The knee*. 194–200.

Clanton, T. O. (1989). Instability of the subtalar joint. *The Orthopedic Clinics of North America, 20:4*, 583–592.

Clement, D. B., Taunton, J. E., & Smart, G. W. (1984). Achilles tendinitis and peritendinitis. Etiology and treatment. *American Journal of Sports Medicine. 12:3*, 179–184.

Cloward, R. B. (1959). Cervical diskography: A contribution to the etiology and mechanism of neck, shoulder and arm pain. *Annals of Surgery, 150:6*, 1052–1064.

Corrigan, B., & Maitland, G. D. (1983). *Practical orthpaedic medicine*. London: Butterworths.

Costello, B. G. (1990). Ligament instability. In J. S. Torg, R. P. Welsh, & R. J. Shephard (Eds.), *Current therapy in sports medicine-2* (pp. 224–229). Toronto and Philadelphia: B.C. Decker Inc.

Cotta, H., & Puhl W. (1978). The pathphysiology of damage ot articular cartilage. In D.E. Hastings (Ed.). *The Knee: Ligaments and articular cartilage injuries* (pp. 15–31). New York: Springer-Verlag.

Courpron, P. (1981). Bone tissue mechanisms underlying osteoporosis. *The Orthopedic Clinics of North America, 12:3*, 513–546.

Creighton, D. S., & Olson, K. L. (1987). Evaluation of range of motion of the first metatarsophalangeal joint in runners with plantar fasciitis. *The Journal of Orthopaedic and Sports Physical Therapy, 8:7*, 357–361.

Curwin, S., & Stanish W. D. (1984). *Tendinitis: Its etiology and treatment*. Lexington: The Collamore Press.

Cyriax, J. (1971). *Cervical spondylosis*. London: Butterworths.

Cyriax, J. (1982). *Textbook of orthpaedic medicine. Volume one. Diagnosis of soft tissue lesions* (8th ed.). London: Bailliere Tindall.

Cyriax, J. (1984). *Textbook of orthpaedic medicine. Volume two. Treatment by manipulation, massage and injection* (11th ed.). London: Bailliere Tindall.

Dandy, D. J. (1986). Arthroscopy in the treatment of young patients with anterior knee pain. *The Orthopedic Clinics of North America, 17:2*, 221–230.

Denis, F. (1988). Cotrel-Dubousset instrumentation in the treatment of idiopathic scoliosis. *The Orthopedic Clinics of North America, 19:2*, 291–311.

Dias, J. J., & Gregg, P. J. (1991). Acromioclavicular joint injuries in sport. Recommendations for treatment. *Sports Medicine, 11*, 125–132.

Donatelli, R. (1990). *The biomechanics of the foot and ankle*. Philadelphia: F. A. Davis Company.

Dovelle, S., & Heeter, P. K. (1989). The Washington regimen: Rehabilitation of the hand following flexor tendon injuries. *Physical Therapy*, 69:12, 1034–1040.

Downs, J., & Twomey, L. (1979). The whiplash syndrome. *Australian Journal of Physiotherapy, 25*, 233–241.

Doxey, G. E. (1987). Calcaneal pain: A review of various disorders. *The Journal of Orthopaedic and Sports Physical Therapy, 9:1*, 25–32.

Duran, R. J., Houser, R. G., Coleman, C. R., & Stover, M. G. (1984). Management of flexor tendon lacerations in zone 2 using controlled passive movement postoperatively. In J. M. Hunter, L. H. Schneider, E. J. Mackin, & A. D. Callahan (Eds.), *Rehabilitation of the hand* (2nd ed.), (pp. 273–276). St. Louis and Toronto: The C. V. Mosby Company.

Echternach, J. L., Jr. (1990). Geriatric hip problems. In J. L. Echternach (Ed.), Clinics in physical therapy. *Physical therapy of the hip* (pp. 205–215). New York: Churchill Livingstone.

Edwards, B. C. (1987). Clinical assessment: The use of combined movements in assessment and treatment. In L. T. Twomey & J. R. Taylor (Eds.), *Clinics in physical therapy. Volume 13. Physical therapy of the low back* (pp. 175–197). New York: Churchill Livingstone.

Edwardson, B. M. (1992). *Musculoskeletal assessment. An integrated approach*. San Diego: Singular Publishing Group, Inc.

Ellman, H. (1990). Arthroscopic subacromial decompression. In J. S. Torg, R. P. Welsh, & R. J. Shephard (Eds.), *Current therapy in sports medicine-2* (pp. 377–380). Toronto and Philadelphia: B. C. Decker Inc.

Elvey, R. L. (1979). Brachial plexus lesion tests and the pathoanatomical origin of arm pain. Aspects of manipulative therapy. *International Conference on Manual Therapy* (pp. 105–110). Melbourne: Lincoln Institute of Health Sciences.

Elvey, R.L. (1986). The investigation of arm pain. In G. P. Grieve (Ed.), *Modern manual therapy of the vertebral column* (pp. 530–535). Edinburgh: Churchill Livingstone.

Engle, R. P., & Giesen, D. P. (1991). Anterior cruciate ligament reconstruction rehabilitation. In R. P. Engle (Ed.), *Knee ligament rehabilitation* (pp. 117–134). New York: Churchill Livingstone.

Farfan, H. F. (1973). *Mechanical disorders of the low back*. Philadelphia: Lea & Febiger.

Fauls, D. (1985). General training techniques to warm up and cool down the throwing arm. In B. Zarins, J.R. Andrews, & W.G. Carson (Eds.), *Injuries to the throwing arm* (pp. 266–276). Philadelphia: W.B. Saunders Company.

Fink, E. P., & Welsh, R. P. (1990). "Impingement syndrome." In J. S. Torg, R. P. Welsh, & R. J. Shephard (Eds.), *Current therapy in sports medicine-2* (pp. 370–373). Toronto and Philadelphia: B. C. Decker Inc.

Fisher, R. L. (1986). Conservative treatment of patellofemoral pain. *The Orthopedic Clinics of North America, 17:2*, 269–272.

Foreman, S. M., & Croft, A. C. (1988). *Whiplash injuries. The cervical acceleration/deceleration syndrome.* Baltimore: Williams and Wilkins.

Gartner, J., & Simons, B. (1990). Analysis of deposits in calcifying tendinitis. *Clinical Orthopaedics and Related Research*, 254, 111–120.

Gill, D. M., Corbacio, E. J., & Lauchle, L. E. (1991). Anatomy of the knee. In R. P. Engle (Ed.), *Knee ligament rehabilitation* (pp. 1–16). New York: Churchill Livingstone.

Gollehon, D. L., Warren, R. F., & Wickiewicz, T.L. (1985). Acute repairs of the anterior cruciate ligament—past and present. *The Orthopedic Clinics of North America, 16:1*, 111–125.

Gramse, R. R., Sinaki, M., & Ilstrup, D. M. (1980). Lumbar spondylolisthesis. A rational approach to conservative treatment. *Mayo Clinic Proceedings, 55*, 681–686.

Grant, R. (1988). Dizziness testing and manipulation of the cervical spine. In R. Grant (Ed.), Clinics in physical therapy, Vol. 17, *Physical therapy of the cervical and thoracic spine* (pp 11–124). New York: Churchill Livingstone.

Grieve, G. P. (1981). *Common vertebral joint problems.* Edinburgh: Churchill Livingstone.

Grieve, G. P. (1982). Neck traction. *Physiotherapy, 68*, 260–265.

Grieve, G. P. 1983). The hip. *Physiotherapy, 69:6*, 196–204.

Hagmeyer, R. H. M., & Van Der Wurff, P. (1987). Transchondral fractures of the talus on an inversion injury of the ankle: A frequently overlooked diagnosis. *The Journal of Orthopaedic and Sports Physical Therapy, 8:7*, 362–367.

Hawkins, R J., & Abrams, J. S. (1987). Impingement syndrome in the absence of rotator cuff tear (stages 1 and 2). *The Orthopedic Clinics of North America, 18:3*, 373–382.

Helfet, A. (1974). *Disorders of the knee.* Philadelphia, Toronto: J.B. Lippincott Co.

Hill, N. A., & Hurst, L. C. (1989). Dupuytren's contracture. *Hand Clinics, 5:3*, 349–357.

Hirsch, S. A., Hirsch, P. J., Hiramoto, H., & Weiss, A. (1988). Whiplash syndrome. Fact or fiction? *The Orthopedic Clinics of North America, 19*, 791–795.

Horner, R. C. (1983). Flexor tendon injuries. In J. A. Boswick, Jr. (Ed.), *Current concepts in hand surgery* (pp. 74–82). Philadelphia: Lea & Febiger.

Howard, L. D., Jr. (1959). Dupuytren's contracture; A guide to management. *Clinical Orthopaedics, 15*, 118–126.

Howell, J. W. (1987). Evaluation and management of thoracic outlet syndrome. In R. Donatelli (Ed.), *Clinics in physical therapy. Volume 11. Physical therapy of the shoulder* (pp. 133–171). New York: Churchill Livingstone.

Huckstep, R. L. (1978). *A simple guide to trauma.* Edinburgh: Churchill Livingstone.

Hutton, P. A. N. (1985) Ankle lesions. In D.H.R. Jenkins (Ed.), *Ligament injuries and their treatment* (pp. 95–111). Maryland: Aspen Publications.

Insall, J. (1979). "Chondromalacia patellae": Patellar malalignment syndrome. *The Orthopedic Clinics of North America*, 10:1, 117–128.

Irrgang, J. (1988). Associated pathologies. In R. E. Mangine (Ed.), *Clinics in physical therapy. Volume 19. Physical Therapy of the knee* (pp. 57–74). New York: Churchill Livingstone.

Jackson, D. L., & Haglund, B. L. (1992). Tarsal tunnel syndrome in runners. *Sports Medicine, 13:2*, 146–150.

James, S. (1979). Chondromalacia of the patella in the adolescent. In J. C. Kennedy (Ed.), *The injured adolescent knee* (pp. 205–251). Baltimore: Williams & Wilkins.

Jobe, F. W., Moynes, D. B., & Brewster, C. E. (1987). Rehabilitation of shoulder joint instabilities. *Orthpedic Clinics of North America, 18:3*, 473–482.

Jobe, F. W., & Bfadley, J. P. (1990). Ulnar neuritis and ulnar collateral ligament instabilities in overarm throwers. In J. S. Torg, R. P. Welsh, & R. J. Shephard (Eds.), *Current therapy in sports medicine-2* (pp. 419–424). Toronto and Philadelphia: B. C. Decker Inc.

Kaltenborn, F. M. (1989). *Manual mobilization of the extremity joints. Basic examination and treatment techniques* (4th ed.). Oslo: Olaf Norlis Bakhandel Universitetsgaten.

Kapandji, I. A. (1974). *The physiology of the joints. Volume 3. The trunk and the vertebral column.* Edinburgh: Churchill Livingstone.

Kapandji, I. A. (1982). *The physiology of the joints. Volume 1. Upper limb.* Edinburgh: Churchill Livingstone.

Kapandji, I. A. (1987). *The physiology of the joints. Volume 2. Lower limb* (5th ed.). Edinburgh: Churchill Livingstone.

Kaput, M. (1987). Anatomy and biomechanics of the shoulder. In R. Donatelli (Ed.), *Clinics in physical therapy. Volume 11. Physical therapy of the shoulder* (pp. 1–16). New York: Churchill Livingstone.

Kenneally, M., Rubenach, H., & Elvey, R. (1988). The upper limb tension test: The S.L.R. test of the arm. In R. Grant (Ed.), *Clinics in physical therapy. Volume 17. Physical therapy of the cervical and thoracic spine* (pp. 167–194). New York: Churchill Livingstone.

Kessel, L. (1982). *Clinical disorders of the shoulder.* Edinburgh: Churchill Livingstone.

Kick, C. (1962). The tarsal tunnel syndrome. *Journal of Bone and Joint Surgery, 44A*, 180–182.

Kirkaldy-Willis, W. H., & McIvor, G. W. D. (1976). Lumbar spinal stenosis. *Clinical Orthopaedics anid Related Research, 115*, 2–4.

Kirkaldy-Willis, W. H. (1983). *Managing low back pain.* New York: Churchill Livingstone.

Kleerekoper, M., Tolia, K., & Parfitt, A. M. (1981). Nutritional, endocrine and demographic aspects of osteoporosis. *The Orthopedic Clinics of North America, 12:3*, 547–558.

Koop, S. E. (1988). Infantile and juvenile idiopathic scoliosis. *The Orthpedic Clinics of North America, 19:2*, 331–337.

Kosmahl, E. M., & Kosmahl, H. E. (1987). Painful plantar heel, plantar fasciitis and calcaneal spur: Etiology and treatment. *The Journal of Orthopaedic and Sports Physical Therapy, 9:1*, 17–24.

Kramer, J. (1981). *Intervertebral disk diseases: Causes, diagnosis, treatment and prophylaxis*. Chicago and London: Year Book Medical Publishers.

Kramer, P. G. (1986). Patellar malalignment syndrome: Rationale to reduce excessive lateral pressure. *The Journal of Orthopaedic and Sports Physical Therapy, 8:6*, 301–309.

Krejci, V., & Koch, P. (1979). *Muscle and tendon injuries*. Chicago: Year Book Medical Publishers.

Kushner, S., & Reid, D. C. (1984). Medial tarsal tunnel syndrome: A review. *The Journal of Orthopaedic and Sports Physical Therapy, 6:1*, 39–45.

Kushner, S., & Reid, D. C. (1986). Manipulation in the treatment of tennis elbow. *Journal of Orthopaedic and Sports Physical Therapy, 7:5*, 264–272.

Lachmoan, S. (1988). *Soft tissue injuries in sport*. London: Blackwell Scientific Publications.

Lam, S.J.S. (1962). A tarsal tunnel syndrome. *Lancet, 2*, 1354–1355.

Lamy, C., Bazergui, A., Kraus, H., & Farfan, H. F. (1975). The strength of the neural arch and the etiology of spondylolisis. *The Orthopedic Clinics of North America, 6:1*, 215–231.

Lankford, L. L. (1984). Reflex sympathetic dystrophy. In J.M. Hunter, L. H. Schneider, E. J. Mackin, & A. D. Callahan (Eds.), *Rehabilitation of the hand* (2nd ed.), (pp. 509–532). St. Louis and Toronto: The C. V. Mosby Company.

Lassiter, T. E., Jr., Malone, T. R., & Garrett, W. E. (1989). Injury to the lateral ligaments of the ankle. *The Orthopedic Clinics of North America, 20:4*, 629–640.

Lee, D. G. (1986). "Tennis elbow": A manual therapist's perspective. *The Journal of Orthopaedic and Sports Physical Therapy, 8:3*, 134–142.

Lee, D. (1989). *The pelvic girdle. An approach to the examination and treatment of the lumbo-pelvic-hip region*. Edinburgh: Churchill Livingstone.

Lestini, W. F., & Wiesel, S. W. (1989). The pathogenesis of cervical spondylosis. *Clinical Orthopaedics and Related Research, 239*, 69–93.

Le Veau, B. (1977). *Williams & Lissner: Biomechanics of human motion*. Philadelphia: W. B. Saunders Company.

Lohr, J.R., & Uhthoff, H. K. (1990). The microvascular pattern of the supraspinatus tendon. *Clinical Orthopaedics and Related Research, 254*, 35–38.

Lonstein, J. E. (1988). Natural history and school screening for scoliosis. *The Orthopedic Clinics of North America, 19:2*, 227–237.

Lonstein, J. E., & Winter, R. B. (1988). Adolescent idiopathic scoliosis: Nonoperative treatment. *The Orthopedic Clinics of North America, 19:2*, 239–246.

Lotke, P. A. (1991). Soft tissue afflictions. In M.E. Steinberg (Ed.), *The hip and its disorders* (pp. 669–682). Philadelphia: W.B. Saunders Company.

MacConaill, M. A., & Basmajian, J. V. (1969). *Muscles and movements: A basis for human kinesiology*. Baltimore: Williams and Wilkins.

Macnab, I. (1971). The whiplash syndrome. *The Orthopedic Clinics of North America, 2*, 389–403.

Macnab, I. (1975). Cervical spondylosis. *Clinical Orthopaedics and Related Research, 109*, 69–77.

Macnab, I. (1977). *Backache*. Baltimore: Williams and Wilkins.

Macnab, I., & Hastings, D. (1968). Rotator cuff tendinitis. *Canadian Medical Association Journal, 99*, 91–98.

Maigne, R. (1972). *Orthopedic medicine: A new approach to vertebral manipulation.* Springfield, IL: Charles C. Thomas.

Maitland, G. D. (1986). *Vertebral manipulation.* (5th ed.). London: Butterworths.

Maitland, G. D. (1991). *Peripheral manipulation* (3rd ed.). London: Butterworth-Heinemann Ltd.

Malek, M. M., & Mangine, R.E. (1981). Patellofemoral pain syndrome: A comprehensive and conservative approach. *The Journal of Orthopaedic and Sports Physical Therapy, 2:3*, 108–116.

Malick, M. H., & Kasch, M. C. (Eds.). (1984). *Manual on management of specific hand problems.* Series I. Pittsburgh: Aren Publications.

Mangine, R. E., & Price, S. (1988). Innovative approaches to surgery and rehabilitation. In R. E. Mangine (Ed.), *Clinics in physical therapy. Volume 19. Physical therapy of the knee* (pp. 191–219). New York: Churchill Livingstone.

Mann, R. A., Baxter, D. E., & Lutter, L. D. (1981). Running Symposium. *Foot and Ankle, 14*, 190–224.

Mann, R. A. (1989). The great toe. *The Orthopedic Clinics of North America, 20:4*, 519–533.

Marshall, J. J., & Baugher, W. H. (1980). Stability examination of the knee. A simple anatomical approach. *Clinical Orthopaedics and Related Research, 146*, 78–89.

Matsen, F. A. III (1975). Compartmental syndrome: An unified concept. *Clinical Orthopaedics and Related Research, 113*, 8–14.

McConnell, J. (1986). The management of chondromalacia patellae: A long-term solution. *Australian Journal of Physiotherapy, 32:4*, 215–223.

McCullough, N. C. (1986). Non-operative treatment of idiopathic scoliosis using surface electrode stimulation. *Spine 11*, 802–804.

McFarlane, R. M., & Albion, U. (1984). Dupuytren's disease. In J.M. Hunter, L. H. Schneider, E. J. Mackin, & A. D. Callahan (Eds.), *Rehabilitation of the hand* (2nd ed.), (pp. 617–624). St. Louis and Toronto: The C.V. Mosby Company.

McKenzie, R. A. (1981). *The lumbar spine. Mechanical diagnosis and therapy.* Waikanae, New Zealand: Spinal Publications.

McKenzie, R. (1983). *Treat your own neck.* P.O. Box 30–865, Lower Hutt, New Zealand: Spinal Publications.

McKenzie, R. A. (1990). *The cervical and thoracic spine. Mechanical diagnosis and therapy.* P.O. Box 93, Waikanae, New Zealand: Spinal Publications (N.Z.). Limited.

McPoil, T. G., & McGarvey, T. C. (1988). The foot in athletics. In G. C. Hunt (Ed.), *Clinics in physical therapy. Volume 15. Physical therapy of the foot and ankle* (pp. 199–229). New York: Churchill Livingstone.

McRae, R. (1981). *Practical fracture treatment.* Edinburgh: Churchill Livingstone.

Meade, T. D. (1991). Meniscus tears: Diagnosis and treatment. In R. P. Engle (Ed.). *Knee ligament rehabilitation* (pp. 51–58). New York: Churchill Livingstone.

Mooney, V., & Robertson, J. (1976). The facet syndrome. *Clinical Orthopaedics and Related Research, 115*, 149–156.

Mooney, V. (1983). The syndromes of low back disease. *The Clinics of North America, 14:3*, 505–515.

Mooney, V. (1987). Where is the pain coming from? *Spine, 12:8*, 754–759.

Moore, K. L. (1980). *Clinically oriented anatomy*. Baltimore, London: Williams and Wilkins.

Moore, R. E., & Friedman, R.J. (1989). Current concepts in pathophysiology and diagnosis of compartmental syndromes. *Journal of Emergency Medicine, 7*, 652–662.

Neer, C. S. II (1972). Anterior acromioplasty for the chronic impingement syndrome in the shoulder. *Journal of Bone and Joint Surgery, 54A*, 41–50.

Neer, C. S. II, & Welsh, R. P. (1977). The shoulder in sports. *The Orthopedic Clinics of North America, 8:3*, 583–591.

Neer, C. S. II (1983). Impingement lesions. *Clinical Orthopaedics and Related Research, 173*, 70–77.

Netter, F. H. (1989). *Atlas of human anatomy*. Summit, N.J.: CIBA-GEIGY Corporation.

Neumann, D. A., & Cook, T. M. (1985). Effect of load and carrying position on the electromyographic activity of the gluteus medius muscle during walking. *Physical Therapy, 65:3*, 305–311.

Neviaser, R. J., (1987a). Injuries to the clavicle and acromioclavicular joint. *The Orthopedic Clinics of North America, 18:3*, 433–438.

Neviaser, R. J. (1987b). Ruptures of the rotator cuff. *The Orthopedic Clinics of North America, 18:3*, 387–394.

Neviasar, T. J. (1987a). The role of the biceps tendon in the impingement syndrome. *The Orthopedic Clinics of North America, 18:3*, 383–386.

Neviaser, T. J. (1987b). Adhesive capsulitis. *The Orthopedic Clinics of North America, 18:3*, 439–444.

Neviaser, R. J., & Neviaser, T.J. (1990). Observations on impingement. *Clinical Orthopaedics and Related Research, 254*, 60–63.

Nirschl, R. P. (1973). Tennis elbow. *The Orthopedic Clinics of North America, 1:3*, 787-799.

Nofthall, F. (1990). Patellofemoral dysfunction. In J. S. Torg, R. P. Welsh, & R. J. Shephard (Eds.), *Current therapy in sports medicine-2* (pp. 275–277). Toronto and Philadelphia: B. C. Decker Inc.

Nordin, M., & Frankel, V. H. (1989). *Basic biomechanics of the musculoskeletal system* (2nd ed.). Philadelphia: Lea & Febiger.

Noyes, F. R., Grood, E. S., Butler, D. L., & Malek, M. (1980). Clinical laxity tests and functional stability of the knee: Biomechanical concepts. *Clinical Orthopaedics and Related Research, 146*, 84–89.

Oatis, C. A. (1988). Biomechanics of the foot and ankle under static conditions. *Physical Therapy, 68:12*, 1815–1812.

Oatis, C. A. (1990). Biomechanics of the hip. In J. L. Echternach (Ed.). *Clinics in physical therapy. Physical therapy of the hip* (pp. 37–50). New York: Churchill Livingstone.

O'Brien, S. J., Warren, R. F., & Schwartz, E. (1987). Anterior shoulder instability. *The Orthopedic Clinics of North America, 18:3*, 395-408.

Ogilvie, J. W., & Sherman, J. (1987). Spondylosis in Scheuermann's disease. *Spine, 12:3*, 251–253.

Outerbridge, R. E. (1961). The etiology of chondromalacia patellae. *Journal of Bone and Joint Surgery, 43B*, 752–757.

Outerbridge, R. E., & Dunlop, J. A. Y. 1975). The problem of chondromalacia patellae. *Clinical Orthopaedics and Related Research, 110*, 177–196.

Patel, D. (1978). Arthroscopy of the plica—synovial folds and their significance. *American Journal of Sports Medicine, 6:5*, 217–225.

Patel, D. (1986). Plica as a cause of anterior knee pain. *The Orthopedic Clinics of North America, 17:2*, 273–279.

Patte, D. (1990). Classification of rotator cuff lesions. *Clinical Orthopaedics and Related Research, 254*, 81–86.

Paulos, L. E., Noyes, F. R., Grood, E., & Butler, D. L. (1981). Knee rehabilitation after anterior cruciate ligament reconstruction and repair. *American Journal of Sports Medicine, 9*, 140–147.

Peterson, L., & Renstrom, P. (1986). *Sports injuries. Their prevention and treatment*. Chicago: Year Book Medical Publishers Inc.

Porter, R.W. (1987). Spinal stenosis in the central and root canal. In M. I. V. Jayson (Ed.), *The lumbar spine and back pain* (pp. 383–400). Edinburgh: Churchill Livingstone.

Pryse-Phillips, W., & Murray, R. J. (1982). *Essential neurology* (2nd ed.). New York: Medical Examination Publishing Co.

Rahlmann, J. F. (1987). Mechanism of intervertebral joint fixation: A literature review. *Journal of Manipulative and Physiological Therapeutics, 10:4*, 177–185.

Rask, M. (1977). Suprascapular nerve entrapment. A report of two cases treated with scapular notch resection. *Clinical Orthopaedics and Related Research, 123*, 73–75.

Rathbun, J. B., & Macnab, I. (1970). The microvascular pattern of the rotator cuff. *Journal of Bone and Joint Surgery, 52B*, 540.

Reichl, M., & Allen, M. J. (1987). Hyperesthesia associated with hyperextension injuries of the neck. *Injury, 18*, 234.

Reid, D. C. (1990). Selected lesions around the talus. In J. S. Torg, P. R. Welsh, & R. J. Shephard (Eds.), *Current therapy in sports medicine-2* (pp. 241–249). Toronto and Philadelphia: B. C. Decker Inc.

Reid, D. C. (1992). *Sports injury assessment and rehabilitation*. New York. Churchill Livingstone.

Renne, J. W. (1975). The iliotibial friction syndrome. *Journal of Bone and Joint Surgery, 57A:8*, 1110–1111.

Rosenberg, L. S., & Sherman, M. G. (1992). Meniscal injury in the anterior deficient knee. A rationale for clinical decision making. *Sports Medicine, 13:6*, 423–432.

Rowe, C. R. (1990). Anterior glenohumeral subluxation/dislocation: The Bankart procedure. In J.S. Torg, R. P. Welsh, & R. J. Shephard (Eds.), *Current therapy in sports medicine-2* (pp. 399–404). Toronto and Philadelphia: B.C. Decker Inc.

Rusche, K., & Mangine, R.E. (1988). Pathomechanics of injury to the patellofemoral and tibiofemoral joint. In R.E. Mangine (Ed.), *Clinics in physical therapy. Volume 19. Physical therapy of the knee* (pp. 31–56). New York: Churchill Livingstone.

Salter, R. B. (1983). *Textbook of disorders and injuries of the musculoskeletal system* (2nd ed.). Baltimore: Williams and Wilkins.

Saunders, H. D. (1979). Classification of musculoskeletal spinal conditions. *The Journal of Orthopaedic and Sports Physical Therapy, 1:1*, 3–15.

Schaberg, J. E., Harper, M. C., & Allen, W. C. (1984). The snapping hip syndrome. *The American Journal of Sports Medicine, 12:5*, 361–365.

Schwartz, E., Warren, R. F., O'Brien, S. J., & Fronek, J. (1987). Posterior shoulder instability. *The Orthopedic Clinics of North America, 18:3*, 409–419.

Seto, J. L., Brewster, C. E., Lombardo, S. J., & Tibone, J. E. (1989). Rehabilitation of the knee after anterior cruciate ligament reconstruction. *The Journal of Orthopedic and Sports Physical Therapy, 11:1*, 8–18.

Shelbourne, K. D., & Nitz, P. (1990). Accelerated rehabilitation after A. C.L. reconstruction. *American Journal of Sports Medicine, 18:3*, 292–299.

Shelokov, A. P. (1991). Evaluation, Diagnosis and initial treatment of cervical disease. *Spine: State of the Art Reviews, 5*, 167–176.

Silverman, B. J., & Greenbarg, P. E. (1988). Idiopathic scoliosis posterior spine fusion with Harrington rod and sublaminar wiring. *The Orthopedic Clinics of North America, 19:2*, 269–280.

Siwek, C. W. (1990). Quadriceps and patellar tendon ruptures. In J. S. Torg, R. P. Welsh, & R. J. Shephard (Eds.), *Current therapy in sports medicine-2* (pp. 277–284). Toronto and Philadelphia: B. C. Decker Inc.

Skurja, M., & Monlux, J. H. (1985). Case studies: The suprascapular nerve and shoulder dysfunction. *The Journal of Orthopaedic and Sports Physical Therapy, 6*, 254–258.

Smith, K. F. (1979). The thoracic outlet syndrome: a protocol of treatment. *The Journal of Orthopaedic and Sports Physical Therapy, 1:2*, 89–99.

Soderberg, G. L. (1986). *Kinesiology. Application ot pathological motion.* Baltimore: Williams and Wilkins.

Sprague, R. B. (1983). The acute cervical joint lock. *Physical Therapy, 63:9*, 1439–1444.

Steindler, A. (1955). *Kinesiology of the human body under normal and pathological conditions.* Springfield: Charles C. Thomas.

Stewart, M. J. (1985). The acromioclavicular joint in the throwing arm. In B. Zarins, J. R. Andrews, & W .G. Carson, Jr. (Eds.), *Injuries to the throwing arm* (pp. 128–143). Philadelphia and Toronto: W.B. Saunders.

Stormont, D. M., Morrey, B. F., An, K.-N., & Cass, J. R. (1985). Stability of the loaded ankle. Relation between articular restraint and primary and secondary static restraints. *American Journal of Sports Medicine, 13:5*, 295–300.

Subotnik, S. I. (1981). Limb length discrepancies of the lower extremity (the short leg syndrome). *The Journal of Orthopaedic and Sports Physical Therapy, 3:1*, 11–16.

Sullivan, J. M. (1990). Rupture of the achilles tendon. In J. S. Torg, R. P. Walsh, & R. J. Shephard (Eds.), *Current therapy in sports medicine-2* (pp. 255–258). Toronto and Philadelphia: B.C. Decker Inc.

Terry, G. C., Hughston, J. C., & Norwood, L. A. (1986). The anatomy of the iliopatellar band and iliotibial tract. *American Journal of Sports Medicine, 14:1*, 39–45.

Threlkeld, A. J., & Currier, D. P. (1988). Osteoarthritis: Effects on synovial joint tissues. *Physical Therapy, 68:3*, 364–370.

Tiidus, P. M. (1990). Exercise and muscle soreness. In J. S. Torg, R. P. Welsh, & R. J. Shephard (Eds.), *Current therapy in sports medicine-2* (pp. 88–92). Toronto, Philadelphia: B.C. Decker Inc.

Torg, J. S. (1990). Plantar fasciiti. In J. S. Torg, R. P. Welsh, & R. J. Shephard (Eds.), *Current therapy in sports medicine-2* (pp. 199–201). Toronto and Philadelphia: B.C. Decker Inc.

Travell, J. G., & Simons, D. G. (1983). *Myofascial pain and dysfunction. The trigger point manual.* Baltimore: Williams and Wilkins.

Trott, P. H., Grant, R., & Maitland, G. D. (1987). Manipulative therapy for the low lumbar spine: Technique selection and application to some syndromes. In L. T. Twomey & J.R. Taylor (Eds.), *Clinics in physical therapy. Volume 13. Physical therapy of the low back* (pp. 199–224). New York: Churchill Livingstone.

Troup, J. D. G. (1976). Mechanical factors in spondylolisthesis and spondylolisis. *Clinical Orthopaedics and Related Research, 117*, 59–67.

Tullos, H. S., & Bryan, W. J. (1985). Functional anatomy of the elbow. In B. Zarins, J. R. Andrews, & W. G. Carson (Eds.), *Injuries to the throwing arm* (pp. 191–200). Philadelphia: W.B. Saunders Company.

Tullos, H.S., & King, J.W., (1973). Throwing mechanism in sports. *The Orthopedic Clinics of North America, 4:3*, 709–720.

Turek, S. L. (1984). *Orthopaedics: Principles and their application. Volume 2.* (4th ed.). Philadelphia: J.B. Lippincott.

van Dam, B .E., Bradford, D. S., Lonstein, J. E., Moe, J. H., Ogilvie, J. W., & Winter, R. B. (1987). Adult idiopathic scoliosis treated by posterior spinal fusion and Harrington instrumentation. *Spine, 12:1*, 32–36.

Vernon-Roberts, B. (1987). Pathology of intervertebral discs and apophyseal joints. In M. I. V. Jayson (Ed.), *The lumbar spine and back pain* (3rd ed.), (pp. 37–55). Edinburgh: Churchill Livingstone.

Wadsworth, C. T., Nielsoen, D. H., Burns, L. T., Krull, J. D., & Thompson, C. G. (1989). Effect of the counterforce armband on wrist extension and grip strength and pain in subjects with tennis elbow. *Journal of Orthopaedic and Sports Physical Therapy, 11:5*, 192–197.

Warwick, R., & Williams, P. L. (Eds.). (1973). *Gray's anatomy* (35th ed.). Edinburgh: Longman Group Ltd.

Wells, P. (1982). Cervical dysfunction and shoulder problems. *Physiotherapy, 68*, 66–73.

Wells, R. (1985). Suprascapular nerve entrapment. In B. Zarins, J. R. Andrews, & W .G. Carson, Jr. (Eds.), *Injuries to the throwing arm* (pp. 173–175). Philadelphia, Toronto: W.B. Saunders.

Welsh, R. P. (1990). Metatarsalgia and other common problems. In J.S. Torg, R. P. Welsh, & R. J. Shephard (Eds.), *Current therapy in sports medicine-2* (pp. 185–189). Toronto and Philadelphia: B. C. Decker Inc.

Welsh, R. P., & Huffer, B. R. (1990). Disorders Affecting tendon structures. In J. S. Torg, R. P. Welsh, & R. J. Shephard (Eds.), *Current therapy in sports medicine-2* (pp. 224–229). Toronto and Philadelphia: B. C. Decker Inc.

Welsh, R. P., & Hutton, C. (1990a). Patellofemoral arthralgia, patellar instability, and chondromalacia patella. In J. S. Torg, R. P. Welsh, & R. J. Shephard (Eds.), *Current therapy in sports medicine-2* (pp. 262–266). Toronto and Philadelphia: B. C. Decker Inc.

Welsh, R. P., & Hutton, C. (1990b). Periarticular overuse syndromes. In J. S. Torg, R.P. Welsh, & R. J. Shephard (Eds.), *Current therapy in sports medicine-2* (pp. 259–262). Toronto and Philadelphia: B.C. Decker Inc.

White III, A. A., & Panjabi, M. M. (1978). *Clinical biomechanics of the spine.* Philadelphia: J. B. Lippincott Company.

Wiltse, L. L., Kirkaldy-Willis, W. H., & McIvor, G. W. D. (1976). The treatment of spinal stenosis. *Clinical Orthopaedics and Related Research, 115,* 83–91.

Winter, R. B., Lonstein, J. E., & Denis, F. (1988). Pain pattern in adult scoliosis. *The Orthopedic Clinics of North America, 19:2,* 339–345.

Wright, C. S. (1990). Overuse syndromes. In J. S. Torg, R. P. Welsh, & R. J. Shephard (Eds.), *Current therapy in sports medicine-2* (pp. 425–426). Toronto and Philadelphia: B. C. Decker Inc.

Wyke, B. (1987). The neurology of low back pain. In M. I. V. Jayson (Ed.), *The lumbar spine and back pain* (3rd ed.). Edinburgh: Churchill Livingstone.

Yong-King, K., & Kirkaldy-Willis, W. H. (1983). The pathophysiology of degenerative disease of the lumbar spine. *The Orthopedic Clinics of North America, 14:3,* 491–504.

Zarins, B., & Nemeth, C. A. (1985). Acute injuries in athletes. *The Orthopedic Clinics of North America, 16:2,* 285–302.

Zoltan, D. J., Clancy, W. G., & Keene, J. E. (1986). A new operative approach to snapping hip and refractory trochanteric bursitis in athletes. *The American Journal of Sports Medicine, 14:3,* 201–204.

# Index

jumper's knee, 185
malalignment syndrome, 178–180
patellar subluxation/dislocation,
    183–184
  recurrent, 184
patellar tendon rupture, 185–186
Patient care
  relationship establishment, 9–10
Pelvic disorders, 171
Pelvic region. *See* Hip joint
Posture. *See also* Treatment
  asymmetries, 3
  classification, 3
  defects, 53–54
  poor, habitually, 106
  sitting illustrated, 38
Putti-Platt surgery, 66, 68

Range of motion
  hypomobility, 5
Reduction
  Kocher method, 66
  shoulder dislocation, anterior, 66
  shoulder dislocation, posterior, 68
Reflex sympathetic dystrophy, 97–99
  clinical features, 98–99
  onset mechanism, 98
  treatment, 99
Rehabilitation
  fracture, 273–274
  tibiofemoral joint cruciate ligament
    injury, 204–205
Relaxants, muscle, 28
Rotator cuff tears, 55, 57–60
  acute, 58
  and cervical spine, 60
  chronic, 58–59
  lidocaine, 59
  and suprascapular nerve disorder
    similarity, 73
  surgery, 58, 59–60
  tests, 59
  treatment, 59–60
Runner's syndrome (tibiofemoral joint),
    212–214
Rupture, muscle, 1

Sacral spine. *See* Spine, lumbar/sacral
Sacroiliac joint (SIJ) problems
  injury mechanism, 138
  syndromes, 138–139
  treatment, 139

Scoliosis, 105–115
  classification, 106–107
  differentiation: structural/non-
    structural, 110
  idiopathic, 106–115
    anatomical changes, 110
    brace, Milwaukee, 113
    Cobb method, measuring/monitoring
      curve, 108
    curve measuring/monitoring, 108
    deformity progression, 109–110
    examination, clinical, 111–113
    lateral electrical surface stimulation
      (LESS), 113
    left lumbar curve, 108
    management, 113–115
    measurements, mobility, 112–113
    observational screening, 112
    rib cage changes, 110
    right thoracic curve, 107
    right thoracic/left lumbar curve, 108
    rotation measuring/monitoring,
      108–109
    screening, 111–112
    tests, mobility, 112–113
    thoracolumbar curve, 107–108
    vertebrae changes, 110
    X-ray rotation measuring/monitor-
      ing, 108–109
  myopathic, 107
  neuropathic, 107
  non-structural, 106
  osteopathic, 107
  structural, 106–115
    cardiorespiratory insufficiency, 111
    complications, 111
    muscle, abnormal functioning, 111
    pain, 111
Sedatives, 137
Shortening, adaptive. *See* Contracture
Shoulder complex. *See also* individual
      problems
  anatomy, 48, 49
  aromioclavicular (AC) joint injuries,
    48–52
  bursitis, 60
  calcified supraspinatus tendon, 60
  and cervical spine involvement
    differentiation, 63
  and cervical spine pain relationship,
    48
  functional aspects, 47

By the same author

*Musculoskeletal Assessment*
*An Integrated Approach*

Singular Publishing Group, Inc.
1992

# MUSCULOSKELETAL DISORDERS
## COMMON PROBLEMS